Essentials in Piezosurgery
Clinical Advantages in Dentistry

Tomaso Vercellotti

...to Margherita, Giuppy, Anna and Nicola.

This book is dedicated to all Surgeons
who deal with Piezoelectric Bone Surgery.

ESSENTIALS
IN PIEZOSURGERY
Clinical Advantages in Dentistry

Tomaso Vercellotti

Milan, Berlin, Chicago, London, Tokyo, Barcelona, Beijing, Istanbul, Moscow, New Delhi, Paris, Prague, São Paulo, and Warsaw

Title of the original version:
Piezosurgery. Elementi Essenziali
Vantaggi clinici in Odontoiatria
Published in 2009 by Quintessenza Edizioni

© 2009 Quintessenza Edizioni
Via Ciro Menotti, 65 - 20017 (Milano)
www.quintessenzaedizioni.it

Vercellotti, Tomaso
Essentials in piezosurgery: clinical advantages in dentistry
ISBN-13: 978185097100

Clinical content: Prof. Tomaso Vercellotti
Illustrations: Anna Vercellotti, Graphic Designer,
        Piezosurgery Academy, Sestri Levante - Italy
Graphic design: Anna Vercellotti, Graphic Designer,
        Piezosurgery Academy, Sestri Levante – Italy
Production: Juliane Richter, Quintessenz Verlags-GmbH,
        Germany

Printed in Italy
ISBN: 978-1-85097-190-0

The content provided in the book Essentials in Piezosurgery – Clinical Advantages of the Use of Ultrasonic Bone Cutting Technology in Dentistry is for demonstration purposes and intended as a brief presentation of the basic concepts of piezoelectric bone surgery. It is also intended to outline the primary clinical benefits of using Mectron-Piezosurgery® technology to improve techniques in orthodontic surgery.

In addition, a preview of the new technique of implant site preparation using ultrasound is presented. An exclusive illustration and summary of the surgical protocol is provided and not the underlying scientific and clinical research.

The reader is referred to the soon-to-be-published book "The Piezoelectric Bone Surgery: A New Paradigm" (written by Tomaso Vercellotti MD, DDS, and published by Quintessence) for insight on each scientific, technological and clinical aspect of piezoelectric bone surgery and for details on the surgical protocol of each technique and for how to use the surgical instruments correctly.

This book, Essentials in Pezosurgery - Clinical Advantages of the Use of Ultrasonic Bone Cutting Technology in Dentistry, should not be considered sufficient for correct clinical application of the techniques outlined.

Foreword

There are infrequent innovations that result in paradigm shifts in the surgical armamentarium for intraoral surgical procedures. Piezosurgery offers distinct advantages to the surgeon as it allows for finite bone incisions with minimal invasiveness and a hemostatic field of vision that significantly reduces the thrust to soft tissues, ie, nerves and blood vessels adjacent to the treatment arena. Equally significant is a quieter, less traumatic experience for the patient that has the potential to reduce postsurgical swelling and discomfort compared to many traditional methods, as it achieves optimal healing.

This exacting atlas of surgical applications presents each surgical technique in a step-by-step manner, demonstrating the surgery and clinical advantages over traditional techniques. Illustrations, diagrams and photographs provide the cutting characteristics that simplify the complexity of intraoral surgical procedures.

It provides the reader an opportunity to visualize a variety of applications and serves as a surgical guide that can be immediately implemented for patient care. It is particularly valuable for procedures that enhance localized edentulous ridges for the purpose of placing dental implants. A distinct value is recognized when performing an osteotomy to lift the maxillary sinus floor, because it will not endanger the Schneiderian membrane, as it stops when encountering soft tissue if properly applied. This results in an intact fold or receptacle to reuse the osteopromotive materials. Thin ridges can be expanded and spread to sufficient dimensions to accept implant dimensions, or intraoral autogenous block grafts can be harvested to add to the thickness.

Piezosurgery offers the clinician the opportunity to perform difficult extractions and to preserve surrounding thin buccal plates in the esthetic zone. These procedures are useful when removing damaged roots without elevators and to section ankylosed or impacted teeth in a precise fashion.

Piezosurgery enables the periodontist to perform osteoplasty, ostectomy and root planing without the noise of conventional handpieces and manual curettes, which are annoying to patients. It is valuable for crown lengthening procedures as well as regenerative efforts.

Exciting recent additions include the preparation of corticotomies to enhance tooth movement in orthodontics and implant site preparation. An upcoming textbook entitled "The Piezoelectric Bone Surgery: A New Paradigm" will expand the opportunity for readers to further their knowledge in these procedures beyond this atlas.

Myron Nevins, DDS

Preface

"Essentials in Piezosurgery" contains a summary of all the elements needed to gain insight into the clinical benefits of piezoelectric bone surgery in dentistry, implantology and oral surgery.

Each surgical technique is presented in a technique-specific manner, showing the surgical, intraoperative, and clinical advantages over traditional techniques.
Illustrations, diagrams, and photographs show the cutting characteristics that make it possible to simplify the complexity of advanced surgery, thus reducing surgical risks and accelerating healing mechanisms. The result is to achieve the highest level of treatment effectiveness with the lowest amount of discomfort for the patient.

The clinical advantages of using piezosurgery over traditional instruments are presented for tooth extraction, ridge expansion, sinus lift, bone grafting, and clinical crown lengthening.

"Essentials in Piezosurgery" also introduces, for the first time in the world, the new technique for ultrasonic implant site preparation and orthodontic microsurgery.

This publication also presents the new bone classification of Tomaso and Giuseppe Vercellotti, which is quantitative and qualitative for each surgical site and enables the highest degree of intraoperatory precision.

The surgical protocol of each technique is presented in photographic sequences in "Essentials in Piezosurgery".

For more in-depth study of the concepts of piezoelectric bone surgery and for learning the step-by-step protocol of each technique, the reader is referred to the soon-to-be-published book "The Piezoelectric Bone Surgery: A New Paradigm", by Tomaso Vercellotti and published by Quintessence. "Essentials in Piezosurgery" is an extract of this book.

Tomaso Vercellotti, MD, DDS

Acknowledgements

I would like to thank all the people who contributed to writing this book.

I would also like to give a special thanks to the following for their invaluable contribution:
- Anna Vercellotti, for the graphics, anatomic and surgical drawings and photographs
- Nicoletta Battilana, for the editing
- Nicolò Cerisola, for writing the section "Technological Perspective"

Summary

SECTION

INTRODUCTION

I

History of the Invention of Piezoelectric Bone Surgery

1.1 Clinical Perspective: The Osteotomy Technique from the Surgical Bur to Piezosurgery

Initial Clinical Idea

In 1997, Tomaso Vercellotti first had the idea to use an ultrasonic device for ablation fitted with a sharpened insert, such as a scalpel blade, to perform periradicular osteotomy to extract an anchylosed root of a maxillary canine. The implant positioned at the moment of the extraction worked perfectly

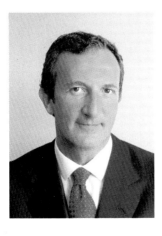

FIG 1-01
Tomaso Vercellotti, the inventor and developer of Piezoelectric Bone Surgery.

and this gave rise to a series of experimental techniques using ultrasound for bone cutting.

Brief History of Ultrasonic Bone Surgery

A thorough literature review[2] revealed that between 1960 and 1981, only five articles were published presenting experimental studies for cutting bone using various instruments, including ultrasound generated by a magnetostrictor.[2,21,22,30,31] These studies had conflicting results, which were not satisfactory for osteotomy due to their lack of surgical efficiency and longer healing time compared to traditional instruments. Eighteen years later, in 1998, Torrella et al.[1] published a technical note describing a bone window osteotomy to lift the maxillary sinus with an ultrasonic piezoelectric ablator.[60]

After testing this technique also for surgery on the maxillary sinus, Tomaso Vercellotti understood its benefits and took note of its drawbacks. He realized that, for instance, with dental extraction, the limited power of normal ultrasonic ablators enabled osteotomy only with thin and sharp inserts. There was a high risk of damaging the sinus membrane, especially since the frame of the bone window made with the osteotomy had such a thin section that it was risky to lift the membrane using manual instruments. This limited power was actually an insurmountable obstacle, especially when attempting to cut a bone wall thicker than one millimeter. Indeed, any attempt to cut thicker bone walls resulted in excessive overheating of the bone itself.

Technological Development of the Mectron-Piezosurgery® Device

In order to overcome the limits of traditional ultrasonic surgery using normal piezoelectric ablators, Tomaso Vercellotti started up a scientific-technological research project with two engineers, his brother Domenico Vercellotti and Fernando Bianchetti, to develop ultrasonic technology that would be ideal for cutting bone.

The experimental phase of lab tests on animal bone yielded the development of an initial prototype called Piezosurgery® right from the beginning. It was found that the higher power over ablators only slightly improved cutting performance and caused excessive overheating of the bone. This problem was solved by designing a frequency over-modulation (US Patent 6,695,847 B2 Mectron Medical Technology), which enables maximum cutting efficiency in both cortical and spongy bone.

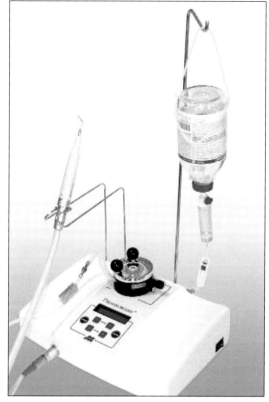

FIG 1-02 1999 - Piezosurgery Dental 1: the first ultrasonic bone surgery device in the world, developed by Mectron S.p.A., Carasco, Italy.

Birth of Piezoelectric Bone Surgery

Tomaso Vercellotti then carried out extensive scientific research in veterinary orthopedic surgery, which enabled him to determine the properties of ultrasonic cutting and obtain the first favorable results of tissue healing.[67]

He immediately understood the clinical importance this new technology could have for all bone surgery; thus, he set up a research group with orthopedists, neurosurgeons, maxillofacial surgeons, and ear-nose-throat surgeons. In addition, encouraged by the research conducted on animals, the author began the clinical

359

Piezoelectric Surgery in Implantology: A Case Report—A New Piezoelectric Ridge Expansion Technique

Tomaso Vercellotti, MD, DDS*

The purpose of this preliminary article is to present a new surgical technique that, thanks to the use of modulated-frequency piezoelectric energy scalpels, permits the expansion of the ridge and the placement of implants in single-stage surgery in positions that were not previously possible with any other method. The technique involves the separation of the vestibular osseous flap from the palatal flap and the immediate positioning of the implant between the 2 cortical walls. The case report illustrates the ridge expansion and positioning of implants step by step in bone of quality 1 to 2 with only 2 to 3 mm of thickness that is maintained for its entire height. To obtain rapid healing, the expansion space that was created for the positioning of the implant was filled, following the concepts of tissue engineering, with bioactive glass synthetic bone graft material as an osteoconductive factor and autogenous platelet-rich plasma as an osteoinductive factor. The site was covered with a platelet-rich plasma membrane. A careful evaluation of the site when reopened after 3 months revealed that the ridge was mineralized and stabilized at a thickness of 5 mm and the implants were osseointegrated. (Int J Periodontics Restorative Dent 2000;20:359–365.)

The presence of a thin edentulous ridge in the maxilla represents a clinical situation in which the positioning of endosseous implants can be complex, and at times impossible, in a single surgical operation. In fact, the minimum thickness of the implant site for the standard method, that is, with preparation of the implant site using burs, is at least 6 mm to permit the positioning of a 3.75-mm implant and the maintenance of a buccal and palatal wall of at least 1 mm.[1-4]

When the thickness of the ridge is reduced to about 4 mm in the most coronal position and the volume increases in the apical direction, preparation of the implant site with burs produces a dehiscence that is generally vestibular and leads to the exposure of several millimeters of the thread of the implant. This dehiscence has to be considered a defect to be treated with additional therapy,[5-8] such as bone grafting and/or guided bone regeneration. This factor reduces the predictability of the treatment because of eventual membrane collapse, exposure, and infection, with incomplete reformation of the bone.[9] When atrophy is

*Private Practice, Genova and Merano, Italy.

Reprint requests: Dr Tomaso Vercellotti, Via XII Ottobre 2/111, 16121 Genova, Italy.

FIG 1-03 The first article in the world introducing piezoelectric bone surgery for ridge expansion.

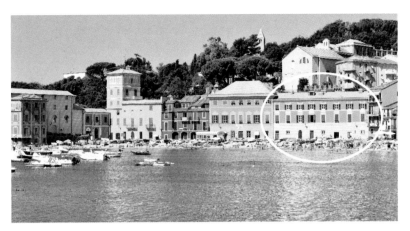

FIG 1-04 Piezosurgery Academy Institute – Baia del Silenzio, Sestri Levante, Italy, location of professional training courses and courses for continuing education.

pioneering phase by developing new surgical protocols in oral, periodontal, and maxillofacial surgery, and by the invention of two new surgery techniques (Ultrasonic Implant Site Preparation and Orthodontic Microsurgery – New-Surgically-Guided Dental Movement). The author realized that a new bone discipline was arising with important clinical and histological features. In 1999, in order to distinguish it from traditional and insufficient ultrasonic bone surgery, he decided to call it "Piezoelectric Bone Surgery".

In 2000, the author published the first article introducing piezoelectric bone surgery in the International Journal of Periondontics and Restorative Dentistry. This publication reported a case of ridge expansion, in which, due to the extreme thinness and mineralization of the edentulous crest, osteotomy would not have been possible with any other surgical instrument.[64,65]

Philosophy of Piezoelectric Bone Surgery

The philosophy behind the development of Piezoelectric Bone Surgery and the entire clinical-scientific research program that led to the development of Mectron–Piezosurgery® is based on two fundamental concepts in bone microsurgery. The first is minimally invasive surgery, which improves tissue healing and reduces discomfort for the patient. The amount of post-operative pain and swelling is always much lower than with traditional techniques.

The second concept is surgical predictability, which increases treatment effectiveness. Indeed, the ease in controlling the instrument during the operation combined with reduced bleeding, the precision of the cut, and the excellent tissue healing make it possible to optimize surgical results even in the most complex anatomical cases.[6,27,50,68,69,70]

Scientific Validation and Dissemination

During the same period, well aware of the responsibility to disclose to the scientific community the benefits and limitations of his invention, the author began an extremely intense period of research and training at several Italian, European and North American universities. This enabled him to develop and fine-tune surgical protocols. Right from the beginning, the scientific research and clinical development of each surgical protocol of piezoelectric bone surgery was made possible thanks to the original technology of Mectron-Piezosurgery®.[7,13,18,47,48,55,61,71,72,75]

This initial scientific, technological, and educational effort produced, directly and indirectly, over 70 publications in leading international magazines and journals dealing with the various aspects and applications of piezoelectric bone surgery in dentistry and maxillofacial surgery.[4,5,9,10,14-16,19,20,24,25,42,43,49,57,62]

Among the most innovative methods developed by the author are the new technique for surgical preparation of the implant site and orthodontic microsurgery.[77]

This small book has been presented to provide a brief description of certain applications and the clinical benefits of piezoelectric bone surgery. Subsequently, a book will be published to provide a thorough and indepth study of all the issues related to this new surgical technique. The book is entitled "The Piezoelectric Bone Surgery: A New Paradigm" (written by Tomaso Vercellotti MD, DDS, Quintessence Publishing).

Learning Piezoelectric Bone Surgery

From a technological standpoint, osteotomy performed with Mectron-Piezosurgery® represents a momentous change from the use of cutters powered by micromotors. The use of bone cutters requires considerable pressure on the handle in order to use the cutting action of the macrovibrations in contact with the bone surface. In contrast, the cut obtained when using ultrasonic microvibrations requires less pressure on the handle, which means acquiring increased surgical control as a result of the right ratio between speed of movement and applied pressure.

In 2005, the Piezosurgery Academy for Advanced Surgical Study was founded to satisfy the increasing demand for training (www.piezosurgeryacademy.com). The goal of the Academy is to introduce operators to the new world of piezoelectric surgery, starting from the basics and on to highly specialized techniques. In particular, all osteotomy and osteoplastic techniques are taught to ensure a high rate of learning.

1.2 Technological Perspective: from Ultrasonic Dental Scaler to Piezosurgery

The Technological Development of Low-frequency Ultrasound: from Scaling to Bone Cutting

Starting in the 1950s, the development of ultrasonic transducers (out of hearing range, ie, higher than 20,000 Hz) attracted increasing interest in several sectors, both industrial and nonindustrial, which considered this "new" form of energy transduction to have important application opportunities.

Among the many sectors, the medical sector is without a doubt the one that over the years has gained the most benefits from developments in this technology. For instance, in the last 20 years, the field of dental scaling has undergone a revolution, passing from the manual use of curettes to the use of sophisticated electromechanical transducers.

The basic technology of these ultrasonic devices uses the piezoelectric phenomenon, an intrinsic property of certain materials. The ultrasound is generated artificially by exploiting the mechanical deformations of quartz or a piezo-ceramic disk.

By applying electrical charges to the face of a quartz plate, the result is crystal compression, and by inverting the direction, expansion results. When the quartz (or piezo-ceramic disk) is placed under an alternating electrical field, it is possible to alternate between compression and expansion of the crystal, thus producing a series of vibrations. When these are conducted through a system (transducer), they generate micrometric movements that

can be used for delicate mechanical operations, such as the removal of calculus.

Another field initially investigated for the generation of ultrasonic vibrations is related to the magnetostriction phenomenon. This is a decisive cause of micrometric deformation in the structure of materials, and in this case, the application of an alternating magnetic field.

However, over the years, the piezoelectric transducer was preferred due to its higher efficiency, mainly because of the fact that the magnetostriction transducer requires dual conversion of energy from electric to magnetic and then from magnetic to mechanical. Some efficiency is lost with every conversion.

At the beginning of the 1980s, Mectron Medical Technology developed and launched an ultrasonic dental scaling device with a highly efficient handle, achieved after carrying out extensive studies on materials and design. For the first time, the transducer had a titanium component and fully exploited the considerable mechanical potential.

The stability of the ultrasonic generation system guaranteed a degree of reliability and mechanical resistance that was unknown in the past. It enabled an extensive range of vibrations and excellent management of thermal dissipation, which is fundamental to achieve a high ratio between electrical energy provided to the handle and mechanical energy as vibrations.

The Mectron-Piezosurgery® Device

Starting from this technological know-how in the field of scaling, Mectron later developed a new ultrasonic instrument for bone surgery. Spurred on by the idea of Tomaso Vercellotti

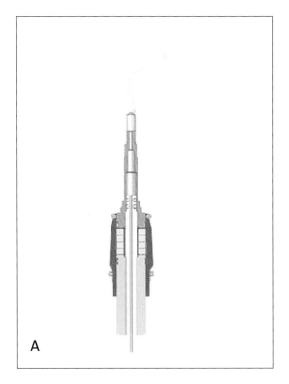

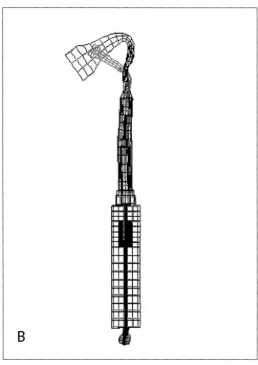

FIG 1-05 From the CAD representation of the transducer with insert OT7 (A) to the FEA analysis of its dynamic behavior (B).

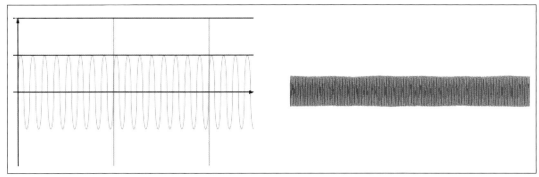

FIG 1-06 Typical form of wave generated by the functioning of a scaling device.

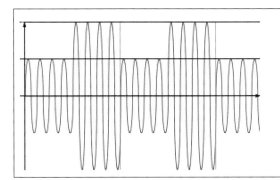

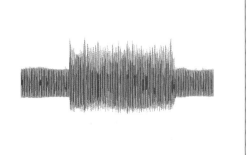

FIG 1-07 The form of wave generated by the functioning of a Mectron-Piezosurgery®; note the over-modulation.

at the end of the 1990s, the first piezoelectric bone surgery instrument was produced and called Mectron-Piezosurgery®.

The close collaboration with Vercellotti led to the development, production, and launching of innovative surgical inserts, each studied and optimized to ensure the highest degree of efficiency according to the clinical need. During this phase, maximum insert performance in terms of mechanical gradient was not pursued, but high level performance of each insert was developed to achieve correct vibration range and direction for specific applications.

The phases of design, research and development took place over a period of years, until the introduction of sophisticated software analysis techniques such as FEA (Finite Element Analysis) helped reduce the planning/prototype development time and enabled the highest degree of optimization of resonant systems.

Additional fine tuning of the already extraordinary properties of the transducer, the absolute innovation of the inserts themselves, and rigorous studies of perfect resonance between the two parties led Mectron to develop an ultrasonic device with extreme mechanical efficiency and clinical effectiveness.

The Mectron-Piezosurgery® device is distinguished by its unique electronic technology. The cutting action, removal and drilling of bone provided by the device have been achieved thanks to a perfect balance between mechanical efficiency and electronic control/handling. Mectron designed a low frequency over-modulation (US Patent 6,695,847 B2) which gives the ultrasonic mechanical vibration its unique nature. The typical resonance frequency of the insert – for Mectron, it is in the range between 24,000 and 29,500 Hz – is coupled with forced oscillation with a frequency ranging between 10 and 60 Hz according to the type of mineralized tissue being operated on. The movement of the insert is comprised of 2 oscillations with the same direction but with different frequencies, resulting in vibrations with optimal energy level to cut bone even at low power levels. Debris is reduced considerably, thus minimizing heat generation on the insert and the substrate.

The "intelligent" electronics of Piezosurgery®, thanks to the integrated feedback system that controls the development of electronic power, also makes it a system able to prevent needless electrical and mechanical stress and to satisfy the needs of the user in a few milliseconds. When the user encounters operational difficulty, the device increases vibration power without altering the feeling of free flow and extreme effectiveness for the user. It is this fact of minimum pressure on the substrate that enhances the properties of Piezosurgery® considering the particular and unique nature of the mechanical vibrations generated.

low-frequency over modulation

resonance frequency of the inserts + forced oscillation

Characteristics of Piezosurgery Surgical Instruments

2

Mectron-Piezosurgery®, developed in collaboration with the author, is the first ultrasonic device dedicated to bone cutting.

The Piezosurgery® unit is composed of the main body, activated with a pedal, a handle, and a number of inserts with different shapes depending on the surgical need.

2.1 Main Body

The main body has a display, an electronic touchpad, a peristaltic pump, one stand for the handle and another to hold the bag containing irrigation fluid.

The interactive touchpad has four keys that enable you to select the feature mode, the specific program, and the flow of cooling fluid. Every command is shown on the display. There are two primary operating modes: BONE mode and ROOT mode.

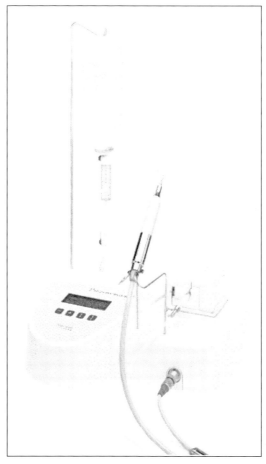

FIG 2-01 Mectron-Piezosurgery® Dental 1: device used to develop piezoelectric bone surgery.

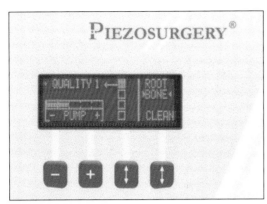

FIG 2-02 Display indicates the Bone Mode, selected depending on bone.

ROOT Mode

The vibrations generated by selecting ROOT mode are characterized by:
- **Average ultrasonic power without frequency over-modulation**
- **Two different programs**
  - **ENDO Program:** a limited level of power provided by applying reduced electrical tension to the transducer, which generates insert oscillation by a few microns. These mechanical microvibrations are optimal for washing out the apical part of the root canal in endodontic surgery.
  - **PERIO Program:** an intermediate level of power between the ENDO program and the BONE program. The ultrasonic wave is transmitted through the transducer in continuous sinusoidal manner characterized by a frequency equal to the resonance frequency of the insert used.

BONE Mode

The vibrations generated by selecting BONE mode are characterized as follows:
- **Extremely high ultrasonic power** compared to Root mode. Its performance is monitored by several sophisticated software and hardware controls.
- **Frequency over-modulation** gives the ultrasonic mechanical vibration its unique nature for cutting different kinds of bone (US Patent 6,695,847 B2). The selection recommended by the author is:
  - **Quality 1:** for cutting the cortical bone or for high-density spongy bone
  - **Quality 3:** for cutting low-density spongy bone
- **SPECIAL Program** was designed with a standard power level slightly lower than the BONE programs and it is characterized by the same frequency over-modulation. The SPECIAL program is dedicated to a limited series of surgical inserts that are particularly thin and delicate. The latter are recommended only for surgeons who have experience using Mectron-Piezosurgery® and would like an extremely thin and effective cut.

For all programs, there is an integrated electronic feedback system that constantly regulates the electrical tension used. This prevents hardware saturation, which can reduce operating efficiency.

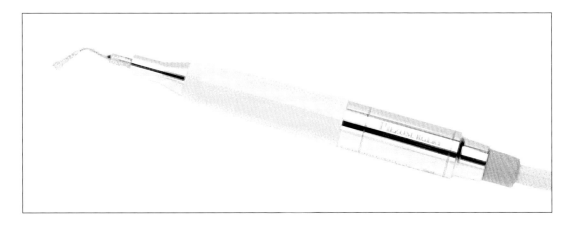

FIG 2-03 Mectron-Piezo-surgery® handle.

2.2 Handle

The cutting action is based on the generation of ultrasonic waves by piezoelectric ceramic disks inside.

These ceramic plates are subjected to an electrical field produced by an external generator and vary their volume to generate ultrasonic vibrations.

These are channeled into the amplifier, which transmits them to the sharp end of the handle. The insert is tightened with a special key for that purpose.

In this manner, the highest degree of efficiency is obtained for the cut and duration of the inserts.

2.3 Inserts

The design and features of all inserts used in Piezoelectric Bone Surgery have been conceived and developed by the author in collaboration with Mectron Medical Technology.

The prototype of each specific insert was developed to satisfy the specific clinical needs of each surgical technique.

All prototypes were then repeatedly tested in the laboratory to study them and improve cutting characteristics, effectiveness, and resistance.

The inserts developed were then used in experimental surgical studies on animals to assess histological results, and in clinical studies to determine operation instructions.

The inserts have been defined and organized according to a dual classification system, taking into consideration morphological-functional and clinical factors. This system helps understand the cutting characteristics and clinical instructions for each insert.

Morphological-functional classification

The morphological description defines the structural properties of the insert, while the functional description outlines the cutting characteristics:

• Sharp - Cutting
• Diamond-coated - Abrasive
• Rounded - Smoothing

Clinical classification

The clinical classification sorts the inserts (sharp, abrasive, smoothing) according to basic surgical technique: osteotomy, osteoplasty, extraction.

- **Osteotomy (OT)**
  OT1 - OT2 - OT3 - OT4 - OT5 - OT6 - OT7 - OT7S4 - OT7S3 - OT8R/L

- **Osteoplasty (OP)**
  OP1 - OP2 - OP3 - OP4 - OP5 - OP6 - OP7

- **Extraction (EX)**
  EX1 - EX2 - EX3

- **Implant site preparation (IM)**
  IM1 (OP5) - IM2A - IM2P - OT4 - IM3A - IM3P

The inserts for basic osteotomy, osteoplasty, and extraction techniques are used in combination with each other and with specific inserts in the surgical protocol for each technique.

- **Periodontal Surgery**
  PS2 - OP5 - OP3 - OP3A - PP1

- **Endodontic Surgery**
  OP3 - PS2 - EN1 - EN2 - OP7

- **Sinus Lift**
  OP3 - OT1 (OP5)- EL1 - EL2 - EL3

- **Ridge Expansion**
  OT7 - OT7S4 - OP5 (IM1) - IM2 - OT4 - IM3

- **Bone Grafting**
  OT7 - OT7S4 - OP1 - OP5

- **Orthodontic Microsurgery**
  OT7S4 - OT7S3

The figures below show the date the first prototype was developed by the company and the date the final version of each insert was produced.

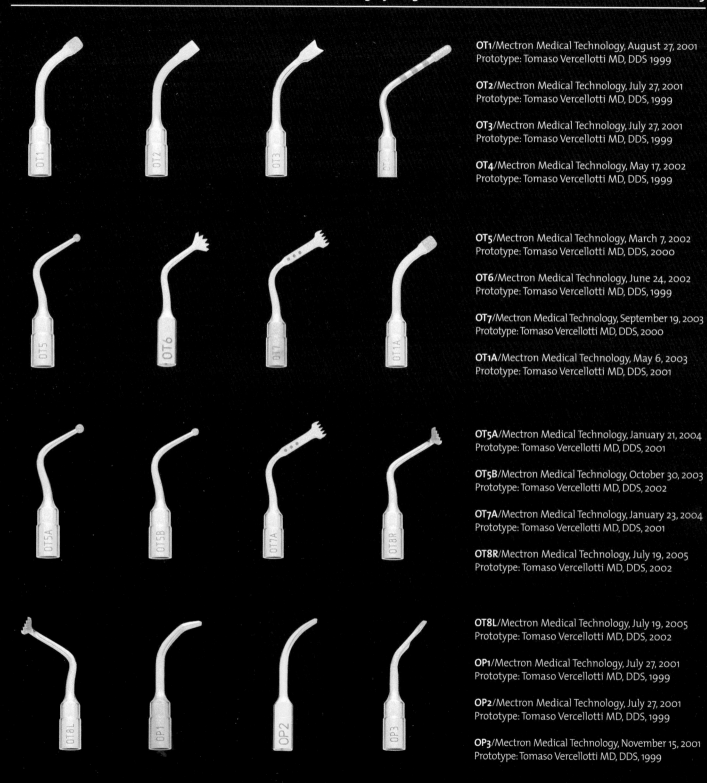

OT1/Mectron Medical Technology, August 27, 2001
Prototype: Tomaso Vercellotti MD, DDS 1999

OT2/Mectron Medical Technology, July 27, 2001
Prototype: Tomaso Vercellotti MD, DDS, 1999

OT3/Mectron Medical Technology, July 27, 2001
Prototype: Tomaso Vercellotti MD, DDS, 1999

OT4/Mectron Medical Technology, May 17, 2002
Prototype: Tomaso Vercellotti MD, DDS, 1999

OT5/Mectron Medical Technology, March 7, 2002
Prototype: Tomaso Vercellotti MD, DDS, 2000

OT6/Mectron Medical Technology, June 24, 2002
Prototype: Tomaso Vercellotti MD, DDS, 1999

OT7/Mectron Medical Technology, September 19, 2003
Prototype: Tomaso Vercellotti MD, DDS, 2000

OT1A/Mectron Medical Technology, May 6, 2003
Prototype: Tomaso Vercellotti MD, DDS, 2001

OT5A/Mectron Medical Technology, January 21, 2004
Prototype: Tomaso Vercellotti MD, DDS, 2001

OT5B/Mectron Medical Technology, October 30, 2003
Prototype: Tomaso Vercellotti MD, DDS, 2002

OT7A/Mectron Medical Technology, January 23, 2004
Prototype: Tomaso Vercellotti MD, DDS, 2001

OT8R/Mectron Medical Technology, July 19, 2005
Prototype: Tomaso Vercellotti MD, DDS, 2002

OT8L/Mectron Medical Technology, July 19, 2005
Prototype: Tomaso Vercellotti MD, DDS, 2002

OP1/Mectron Medical Technology, July 27, 2001
Prototype: Tomaso Vercellotti MD, DDS, 1999

OP2/Mectron Medical Technology, July 27, 2001
Prototype: Tomaso Vercellotti MD, DDS, 1999

OP3/Mectron Medical Technology, November 15, 2001
Prototype: Tomaso Vercellotti MD, DDS, 1999

OP4/Mectron Medical Technology, July 27, 2002
Prototype: Tomaso Vercellotti MD, DDS, 2000

OP5/Mectron Medical Technology, July 1, 2002
Prototype: Tomaso Vercellotti MD, DDS, 2000

OP6/Mectron Medical Technology, June 25, 2002
Prototype: Tomaso Vercellotti MD, DDS, 1999

OP7/Mectron Medical Technology, May 23, 2002
Prototype: Tomaso Vercellotti MD, DDS, 2000

OP6A/Mectron Medical Technology, June 27, 2002
Prototype: Tomaso Vercellotti MD, DDS, 2001

OP3A/Mectron Medical Technology, June 3, 2003
Prototype: Tomaso Vercellotti MD, DDS, 2001

EX1/Mectron Medical Technology, November 15, 2001
Prototype: Tomaso Vercellotti MD, DDS, 1999

EX2/Mectron Medical Technology, November 15, 2001
Prototype: Tomaso Vercellotti MD, DDS, 1999

EX3/Mectron Medical Technology, November 11, 2005
Prototype: Tomaso Vercellotti MD, DDS, 2002

EL1/Mectron Medical Technology, July 23, 2001
Prototype: Tomaso Vercellotti MD, DDS, 1999

EL2/Mectron Medical Technology, July 23, 2001
Prototype: Tomaso Vercellotti MD, DDS, 1999

EL3/Mectron Medical Technology, July 23, 2001
Prototype: Tomaso Vercellotti MD, DDS, 1999

PP1/Mectron Medical Technology, November 8, 2001
Prototype: Tomaso Vercellotti MD, DDS, 1999

PS1/Mectron Medical Technology, November 8, 2001
Prototype: Tomaso Vercellotti MD, DDS, 1999

PS2/Mectron Medical Technology, May 23, 2002
Prototype: Tomaso Vercellotti MD, DDS, 2000

PS6/Mectron Medical Technology, June 26, 2002
Prototype: Mectron, 1999

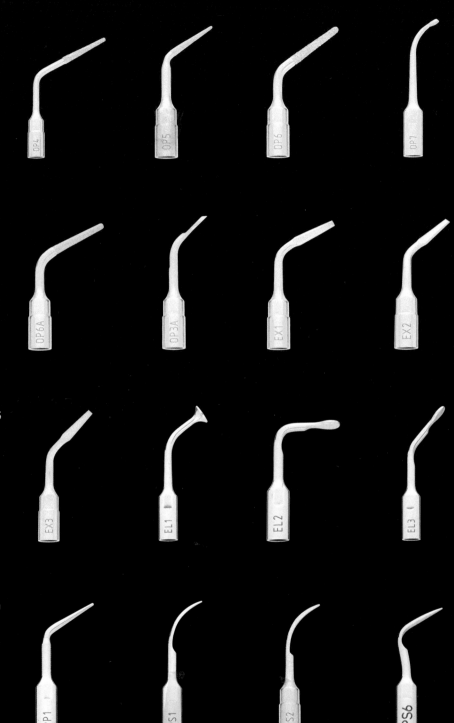

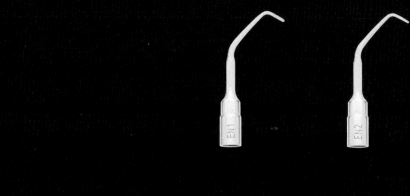

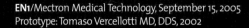

EN1/Mectron Medical Technology, September 15, 2005
Prototype: Tomaso Vercellotti MD, DDS, 2002

EN2/Mectron Medical Technology, September 15, 2005
Prototype: Tomaso Vercellotti MD, DDS, 2002

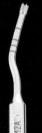
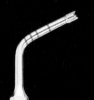
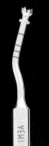
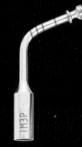

IM 2A/Mectron Medical Technology, February 24, 2007
Prototype: Tomaso Vercellotti MD, DDS, 2003

IM 2P/Mectron Medical Technology, February 24, 2007
Prototype: Tomaso Vercellotti MD, DDS, 2003

IM 3A/Mectron Medical Technology, February 24, 2007
Prototype: Tomaso Vercellotti MD, DDS, 2003

IM 3P/Mectron Medical Technology, February 24, 2007
Prototype: Tomaso Vercellotti MD, DDS, 2003

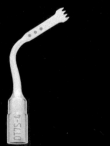
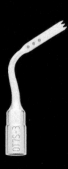

OT7S 4/Mectron medical Technology, September 2008
Prototype: Tomaso Vercellotti MD, DDS, 2006

OT7S 3/Mectron medical Technology, September 2008
Prototype: Tomaso Vercellotti MD, DDS, 2006

NOTE: Steel color insert tips cannot be used
in BONE mode.

SECTION II

TECHNOLOGY AND SURGERY

Clinical Characteristics and Surgical Protocols

3

[handwritten annotations: — precision / — efficiency / — selective / — blood-free surg field / — favourable osseous response / better healing / — less stress / for pt, surgeon, tissue]

3.1 Clinical Characteristics of Piezosurgery Cutting Action

Precise Cutting Action

The cutting precision depends on mechanical microvibrations whose linear oscillation runs from 20 to 80 microns. This microscopic spread provides microsurgical precision to cutting, and the limit depends only on the degree of enlargement used by the operator. In spite of the microscopic linear dimensions of the vibrations, their cutting efficiency is considerable, even with the naked eye, because the frequency is about 30,000 times per second.

Selective Cutting Action

This physical property, which enables better cutting of mineralized tissues than soft tissues, depends on the low frequency of the ultrasonic waves and on the sharpness of the insert used. In the vicinity of delicate soft tissues, such as the sinus membrane or alveolar nerve, it is recommended to finish off cutting

with a diamond coated insert, without intrinsic cutting, which slows down cutting but makes it safer. Indeed, the only effect of accidentally touching soft tissue with a blunt insert is that the heat stops.

Thus, selective cutting is an important clinical characteristic that is very helpful in the proximity of the maxillary sinus and nerve endings.

Some of the benefits of selective cutting in two different anatomical situations, near the maxillary sinus and the alveolar nerve, are described below.

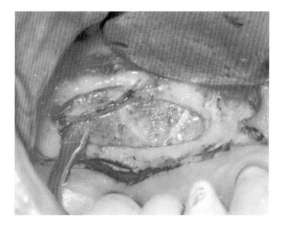

FIG 3-01 Example of selective cut in maxillary sinus surgery: the Piezosurgery® insert respects soft tissues when cutting bone. Notice the vascular formation is intact as well as the Schneiderian membrane after removing the bony window.

• **Sinus membrane preservation**

The literature reveals that osteotomy of the maxillary lateral wall for sinus surgery performed with burs results in puncturing the Schneiderian membrane in 14 to 56% of cases depending on the operator.[8,58,59,80]

Using Mectron-Piezosurgery®, the risk of puncturing the membrane drops considerably, to an average of about 7% on an average learning curve.

In a recent article published by New York University, the authors demonstrated that the percentage of membrane perforation in 100 consecutive cases using Mectron Piezosurgery® drops to 7%, compared to 30% obtained, by the same operators, using burs.[81]

These results are achieved by following a strict surgical protocol, which enables access osteotomy with safety in a very short time.

Not knowing the surgical protocol results in an increased risk of puncturing the membrane, on an average similar to that of burs.[3]

• **Nerve preservation**

The results of experiments performed on animals to examine the risk of neurological damage by accidental surgical contact with a peripheral nerve using Mectron-Piezosurgery® have demonstrated that prolonged contact for 5 seconds provokes permanent neurological consequences in only 10% of animals.[46] It should be remembered that with a bone bur, only 1 second of contact is enough to cut a nerve ending, resulting in total and permanent damage.

Results of clinical studies in orthognathic surgery have demonstrated that the risk of post-operative neurological damage dropped considerably and is not comparable to results obtained using bone burs.[13,41,45]

In any case, the author recommends caution in executing the osteotomy near delicate anatomical areas. This type of operation requires a high degree of skill, and so only proficient surgeons who have received adequate training should perform it.

Intra-operatory Surgical Control

Surgical control of a cutting instrument for bone surgery is decisive to achieve the desired result.

Bone burs need about 2 to 3 kg of pressure on the handle in order to cut. This reduces sensitivity during the operation, and surgical control is critical when working in areas with bone mineralization, particularly in the proximity of delicate anatomical structures such as vascular-nerve structures. Indeed, the cutting action is through macrovibrations generated by the burs.

On the contrary, the cutting action produced by Mectron-Piezosurgery® microvibrations requires a pressure of 500 g. The consequence is that the reduced force applied to the handle and the microvibrations generated by the cutting action increases surgical control, resulting in a reduction of anatomical risks.

Intra-operatory control together with cutting precision has resulted in quick success for Mectron-Piezosurgery®.

Insert Efficiency

All inserts used in Piezoelectric Bone Surgery have been developed by Mectron in close collaboration with Tomaso Vercellotti, who tested each one first in the laboratory and then in the clinic in order to optimize them for every specific need.

These new forms, once unknown in bone surgery, have made it possible to simplify and make safer numerous surgical techniques, as seen in the clinical examples provided.[53]

Bone healing response was studied for the most important inserts in comparison with burs. The result is very fast healing.[78]

Bloodfree Surgical Site

Bone surgery using Mectron-Piezosurgery® is characterized by high visibility during the operation due to the fact that there is no bleeding when cutting.

This is due to the coolant saline solution, which, on contact with the insert vibrating at ultrasonic speed, produces the cavitation phenomenon. This phenomenon consists of the formation of vapor bubbles within the coolant liquid. These bubbles implode, generating a shock wave.

From a clinical standpoint, cavitation results in stopping blood from flowing out of the capillary during cutting.[70]

Bleeding starts again immediately after cutting ends.

Hemostasis is an enormous clinical advantage in many anatomical situations, particularly during extraction processes to remove a fractured apex.

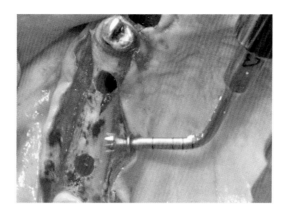

FIG 3-02 Example of excellent intraoperatory visibility. During implant site preparation, there is no bleeding, thanks to cavitation of the coolant liquid (sterile saline solution).

The osteotomy action is generally very quick, so the momentary absence of bleeding means no consequences for tissue healing. It is recommended that excessive washout of the bone surface be avoided, and, if necessary, the osteotomy procedure be interrupted by brief pauses.

Favorable Osseous Response

All histological and biomolecular studies on bone healing in areas where the osteotomy is performed using Mectron-Piezosurgery® demonstrated many more advantages to healing than using bone burs.[56,64,74,78]

In particular, the microscopic test showed that the areas treated lacked the lamellar fragmentation typical of bone burs, lacked pigmentation from overheating, and had vital osteocytes on the osteotomy surfaces.

SEM studies have shown an irregular surface after using the bone bur, a surface covered with bone debris after using a bone saw, and a rough surface, perfectly clean, immediately covered with fibrin when using Mectron-Piezosurgery®.[79]

Histomorphometric studies have shown that in the preparation of the implant site, there are fewer inflammatory cells when using Mectron-Piezosurgery® instead of the twist drill.

In addition, the density of osteoclasts is much higher and bone regeneration takes half the time.

Biomolecular results have shown a notable difference in the concentration of MP4 and TGF-β2, following the use of Mectron-Piezosurgery®. In particular, MP4 and TGF-β2 value in the initial phase of healing were found to be 18.5–19 times higher than those following the use of spiral bur.

In conclusion, studies have begun to provide answers to why healing observed in the clinic after Mectron-Piezosurgery® is much better than when using traditional instruments.

Reduced Operation Stress

Operation stress suffered by the patient from cutting performed with Mectron-Piezosurgery® is less than that when burs are used to extract third molars (University of Padua, Dr. S. Sivolella, unpublished data).

The noise of the device is very similar to that of an ablator, and above all, the microvibrations are much more tolerable than macrovibrations.

A surgeon's stress during the operation is much less than when using a bur, thanks to the precision mentioned above as well as intra-operatory control, respect for soft tissues, operation visibility, and better patient compliance.

The stress on tissues is much less thanks to the better healing response.

3.2 Surgical Protocol for each Technique

The creative route that led the author to develop a specific surgical protocol for every technique is based on strict guidelines.

The starting point is always a clinical idea, conceived to solve a surgical problem, followed by a technological answer that is first tested in vitro, then in vivo, and finally it is used on a patient.

Critical assessment of histological-clinical results makes it possible to optimize materials and methods which are gathered in a file and used to develop the surgical protocol.

Surgical Need

Each surgical technique conceived and developed using Mectron-Piezosurgery® answers a need of the author to overcome the precision and safety limitations of traditional instruments used for bone surgery.

For the first time in the history of Medicine, this has enabled the development of ultrasonic terminals dedicated exclusively to bone cutting, and each one is characterized by the best form for the function desired.

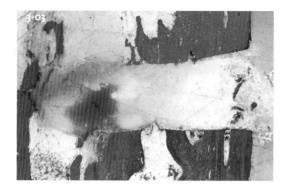

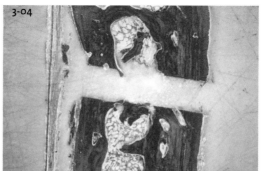

FIG 3-03 Osteotomy produced by 0.9 mm diameter bone bur. Notice the lamellar fragmentation.

FIG 3-04 Osteotomy performed with 0.5 mm OT7. Notice the bone walls remain intact.

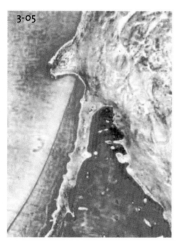

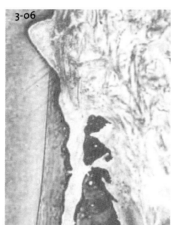

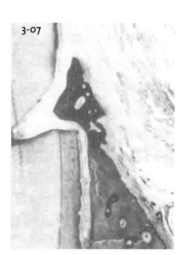

FIG 3-05, 3-06, 3-07 Technique for clinical crown lengthening (experimental study)67
The histological diagrams show the result of bone tissue healing 56 days after the ostectomy

• FIG 3-05 Carbide bur: bone healing nearly reached the lower level of the edge of the intraoperatory mark made on the root surface.
• FIG 3-06 Diamond-coated bur: bone healing is much slower than when the carbide bur is used.
• FIG 3-07 OP3 Piezosurgery: bone healing is excellent and passes the upper end of the intraoperatory mark made on the root surface.

In Vitro Tests on Animal Bone to Evaluate Insert Performance and Effectiveness

After determining the ideal form of the insert for each technique and after overcoming technological issues for fine-tuning, specific laboratory tests were performed on animal bone to achieve the highest degree of surgical efficiency in terms of precision and time. This work made it possible to obtain all the ultrasonic inserts currently used in Piezo-electric Bone Surgery.

The inserts are classified based on their specific function and cutting properties. Insert classes based on function are Osteotomy (OT), Osteoplasty (OP), Extraction (EX) and Implant Site Preparation (IM). Insert classes based on ultrasonic cutting properties, regardless of their function, are Sharp, Smoothing, and Blunt.

FIG 3-08, 3-09, 3-10 Assessment of bone healing in the osteotomy areas 7 days after surgery. The cuts were performed using the most efficient instruments available on the market (2.5x zoom).

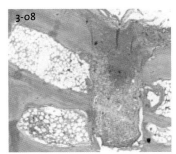

FIG 3-08 Bone bur: the osteotomy area has connective tissue and osteoblast cells for periosteal reaction.

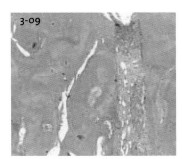

FIG 3-09 Bone saw: the osteotomy area has connective tissue and the inner part has bone fragments with newly-formed bone from periosteal reaction.

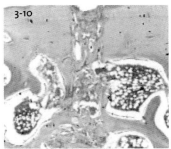

FIG 3-10 Piezosurgery OT7: the osteotomy area is full of newly-formed bone from periosteal reaction and endostyle cells, a clear sign that tissue regeneration is much faster in the first weeks.

FIG 3-11, 3-12, 3-13 Assessment of the morphology of the bone surface with an SEM.

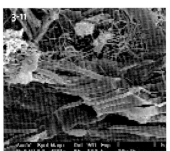

FIG 3-11 Bone bur: the bone surface appears extremely irregular.

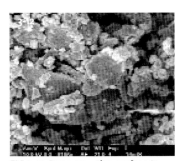

FIG 3-12 Bone saw: the surface is covered with bone debris.

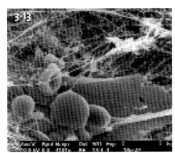

FIG 3-13 Piezosurgery OT7: the surface is microporous, perfectly cleansed, and immediately covered with the fibrin that initiates coagulation, a clear sign of the speed of mechanisms for tissue healing.

Histological Evaluation to Observe Bone Tissue Healing Response

The main inserts for Osteotomy, Osteoplasty, and Implant Site Preparation were tested live through experiments on animals to assess tissue healing response.

These histological and biomolecular studies were carried out by the author over the last 9 years and performed in collaboration with major Italian and North American universities (Orthopedics Department of University of Genoa, Otholaryngology Department of University of Genoa, Periodontal Department of University of Padua, Prosthodontic Department of University of Turin, Periodontal Department of Harvard University, USA). The results achieved demonstrated bone healing response time that is much faster than that after using burs or perforating twist drills.[2,30,31,67,78]

Clinical Pioneering Phase

Once favorable results were achieved from research conducted on animals, the author began the clinical pioneering phase to understand the benefits of using Mectron-Piezosurgery® in odontological surgery. During the first years, the effort was focused on optimizing already existing surgical protocols (Sinus Lift, Ridge Expansion, Bone Grafting) while more recently, new surgical techniques were conceived and developed to greatly improve the state of the art in Dentistry. Indeed, two new techniques have been introduced that enable the development of current orthodontic and implant treatment.

In this book, the technique developed by the author for ultrasonic preparation of the implant site is published for the first time.

Phases of Clinical Studies

Several clinical studies have appeared in the literature starting from initial publications and extensive educational activities conducted by the author. The results of the latter and those presented at several congresses by various speakers have made it possible to define a surgical protocol for each technique.

Surgical Protocol

The current surgical protocol, developed by the author for each technique, not only provides instructions for correct use of Mectron-Piezosurgery®, but it is also a complete guide for correct performance of surgery step by step, from incision of the flap to final suture. This surgical protocol, used successfully in professional training courses, enables beginners to avoid the most common errors and experienced clinicians to accelerate their learning curve.

The surgical protocol specific to each surgical technique is outlined in a dedicated file for easy day-to-day professional use.

These tables have been thoroughly described and annexed in the book "The Piezoelectric Bone Surgery: A New Paradigm" written by Tomaso Vercellotti, soon to be published.

SECTION III

CLINICAL ADVANTAGES
OF PIEZOSURGERY
IN DENTISTRY

Tooth Extraction Techniques

4

Dental extraction is a surgical operation that is necessary when an element cannot be restored with predictable treatment.

The most common causes of dental extraction are advanced periodontal disease, destructive decay, untreated endodontic lesions, and root fractures.

The surgical technique is correct when removal of the root does not cause damage to the alveolar walls and periodontium surface. Surgical difficulty of extraction depends on periodontal anatomy characteristics.

4.1 Anatomical Characteristics and Surgical Techniques

- **Normal Periodontium: Simple Extraction Performed with Manual Instruments**

When there is a normal periodontium, extraction is considered simple and manual instruments are used.

Extraction entails:
- cutting the periodontium surface using a periotome
- displacement of ligament fibers using a lever
- root avulsion from the alveolar bone using forceps

Where there is a normal periodontium, using mechanical or ultrasonic instruments is not recommended, since it is not necessary to cut mineralized tissues to obtain the mobility needed for extraction.

- **Anchylotic Root: Complex Extraction Performed with Mechanical Instruments**

Anchylotic tooth extraction is impossible if the root is not made mobile.

The lever is not able to obtain mobility without fracturing the alveolar walls.

A common technique is to use a bur to perform a periradicular osteotomy to separate the root from the bone and to obtain mobility with the lever.

This technique causes damage to the alveolar walls, thus creating a defect in the implant space.

The technique developed and proposed by the author, using Mectron-Piezosurgery®, entails using an extremely thin insert (Mectron-Piezosurgery® EX1) which cuts away the anchylosis, thereby removing the root surface and maintaining the alveolar walls intact.

4.2 Surgical Protocol of Tooth Extraction using Piezosurgery

The author developed 4 surgical protocols for dental extraction that are able to meet the needs of the anatomical complexity of any periodontal condition:
- anchylotic root
- thin periodontal biotype
- anchylotic root in thin periodontal biotype

Presurgical study of these new extraction techniques will help the operator decide when it is preferable to use a flapless or open-flap extraction technique, above all when assessing aesthetic and reconstructive results. Below are the extraction techniques where using Mectron-Piezosurgery® is particularly beneficial to simplify extraction, provide predictable results for maintaining periodontal tissues intact, and to reduce patient discomfort.

Table 4.1 Clinical Advantages of Using Mectron-Piezosurgery® in Tooth Extraction Techniques

SURGICAL TECHNIQUE	LIMITS OF TRADITIONAL INSTRUMENTS	ADVANTAGES USING PIEZOSURGERY
1. Anchylotic root extraction	The traditional technique using a bur entails a perioradicular osteotomy with removal of alveolar bone. This technique often results in loss of thin buccal bone.	Using the Mectron-Piezosurgery® EX1 insert, anchylosis removal is by removing the root surface while maintaining the integrity of the alveolar bone even when the buccal wall is very thin.
2. Extraction of impacted third molar	After performing the crown resection with the bur, rhizotomy is risky near the lingual cortical bone due to reduced intra-operative sensitivity, which does not always enable the operator to feel whether enamel cutting is complete, with the risk of beginning cortical cutting. When it is necessary to remove a fractured apex, the process is very slow and difficult due to bleeding, which reduces intra-operative visibility. Most of the time it is necessary to use thin suction terminals and make intra-alveolar injections of anesthetic with vasoconstriction.	After beginning the cutting action on the crown with the bur, rhizotomy and root fractioning performed with Mectron-Piezosurgery® (EX OT7S inserts) is very precise and allows the highest degree of intra-operative sensitivity without damaging the alveolar walls. The saline solution's cavitation effect provides hemostasis during the cutting action and gives the operator maximum visibility. In this way, even removal of root fragments of an apex becomes very simple. It is enough to use the tip of the PS2 insert in the endodontic channel so that the vibrations immediately detach the apex from the alveolus. In the event of apex anchylosis, it is possible to use a curette-shaped insert (PS 2, OP5, IM1, EX1S) to perform a perioradicular osteotomy to ease extraction.

SURGICAL TECHNIQUE	LIMITS OF TRADITIONAL INSTRUMENTS	ADVANTAGES USING PIEZOSURGERY
3. Extraction of polyradiculitis tooth, rhizotomy technique	After performing the crown resection with the bur, rhizotomy is risky due to reduced intra-operative sensitivity. Using a bur to remove a polyradiculitis tooth entails the risk of damaging the other roots.	Rhizotomy is necessary for extracting polyradiculitis teeth to preserve alveolar integrity during extraction. With Mectron-Piezosurgery®, the extraction technique is extremely simple and consists of crown resection below the cementum level with OT7S4 and with separation of each root extracted individually. The rhizotomy technique without extraction, using Mectron-Piezosurgery®, is extremely precise and at the end it is possible to perform. osteoplastic remodeling with the diamond insert OP5 to optimize the surface of the emergency root profile.
4. Root fractioning techniques	Root fractioning inside the alveolar is very difficult with the bur and there is the risk of causing major damage to the alveolar walls.	Using Mectron-Piezosurgery®, root fractioning can easily be performed with different techniques using the OT7S3, which enables root fractioning also when the diameter of the alveolar is small.
5. Exposing or extracting impacted teeth	Osteotomy using the bur is difficult due to bleeding and the risk of damaging enamel.	With Mectron-Piezosurgery®, the osteotomy technique to reach the crown of the impacted tooth with insert OP3 makes it possible to keep enamel intact and cavitation gives maximum visibility during the operation.[17] Since there is no bleeding, it is much easier to bond orthodontic brackets. For extraction, the tooth is fractioned as described above.

Ankylotic Root Extraction

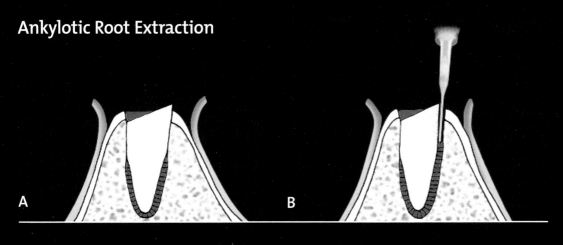

A: Fractured root to be extracted: notice that ankylosis affects the coronal part of the root.

B: The EX1 insert removes the ankylosis by wearing down the root surface without overheating the alveolar bone.

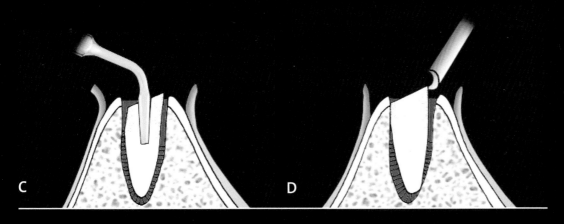

C: Following root osteoplasty, a newly obtained space between root surface and alveolar bone is visible.

D: Using a manual lever, it is possible to smoothen the ligament and obtain mobility.

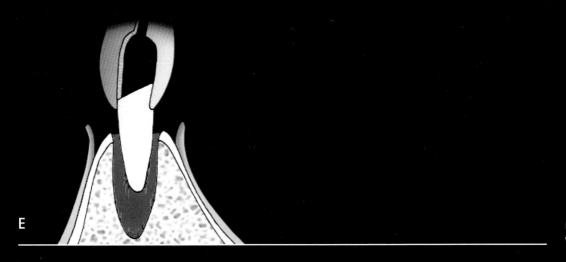

E: Lastly, the root is extracted with forceps.

CASE I

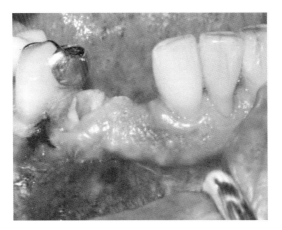
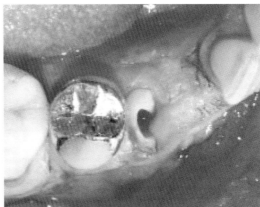

FIG 4-01 Buccal view of the root fracture of the first mandibular right premolar.

FIG 4-02 Occlusal view of the fractured ankylotic root.

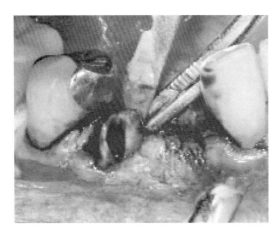
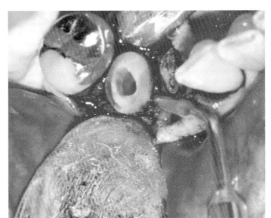

FIG 4-03 Incision with a no. 15 scalpel blade.

FIG 4-04 The EX1 insert removes the ankylosis by wearing down the root surface.

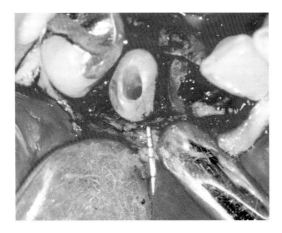
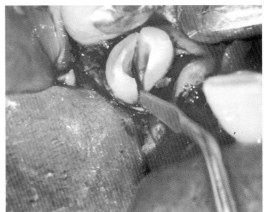

FIG 4-05 Alveolar bone wall thinness is visible.

FIG 4-06 The EX1 insert is used to perform a mesio-distal root resection.

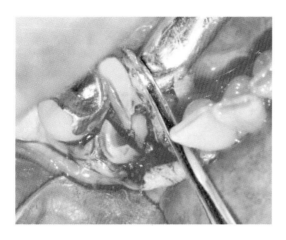

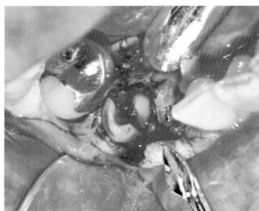

FIG 4-07 The lever force moves the root's lingual portion.

FIG 4-08 Root fragments still attached to the alveolar bone.

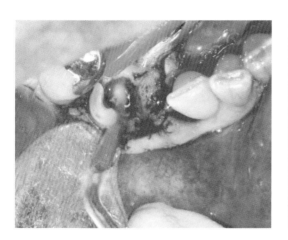

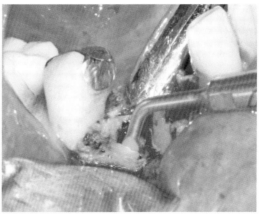

FIG 4-09 The EX1 insert is used to remove the ankylosis.

FIG 4-10 The EX1 goes down the entire length of the anckylosis, concentrating the action only on the root surface.

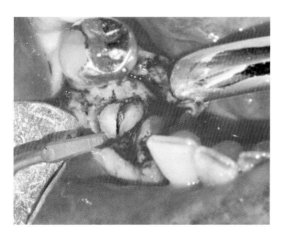

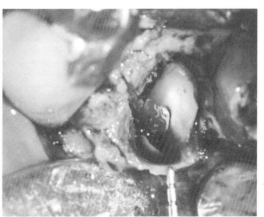

FIG 4-11 Occlusal view of the root osteoplasty technique.

FIG 4-12 The periodontal probe measures the integrity of the buccal cortex where the bone has not been worn down. Thanks to the thickness of the lingual wall, a peri-radicular osteotomy can be performed.

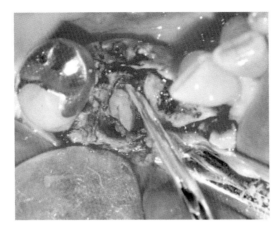

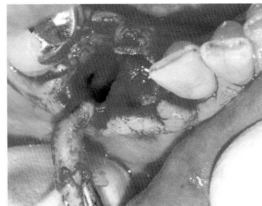

FIG 4-13 Inserting the manual lever loosens the root fragment in the alveolus without jeopardizing the buccal bone crest.

FIG 4-14 After removing the coronal part of the ankylosis, extraction is simply performed.

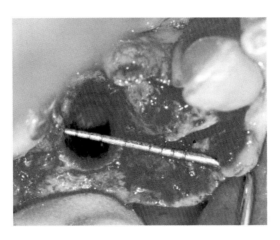

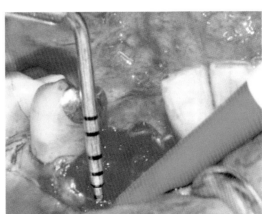

FIG 4-15 Following the extraction, alveolar integrity can be observed, regardless of initial ankylosis severity.

FIG 4-16 Natural alveolar depth is measured.

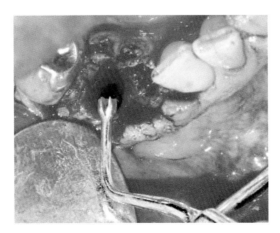

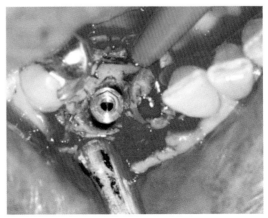

FIG 4-17 The IM2 insert is used to prepare the implant site.

FIG 4-18 Occlusal view of the alveolar-implant interface.

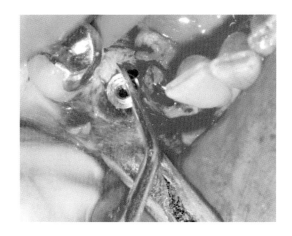
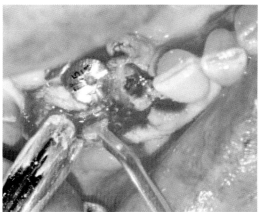

FIG 4-19 The OP3 insert is used to perform a peri-implant osteoplasty

FIG 4-20 The bone chips collected during osteoplasty are used to fill the alveolar-implant interface.

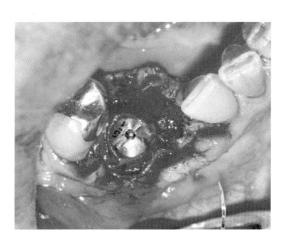
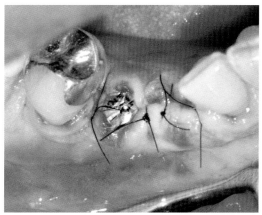

FIG 4-21 The bone chips are stabilized with a resorbable collagen membrane.

FIG 4-22 The suture around the healing post.

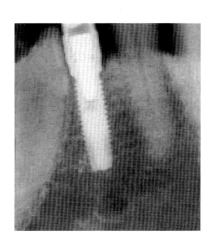

FIG 4-23 Implant radiograph (3 years later).

CASE II

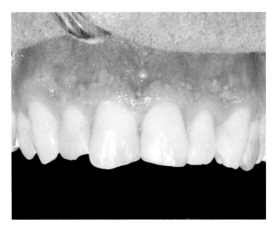
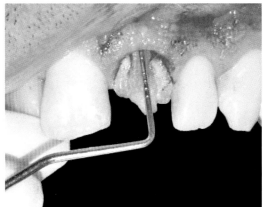

FIG 4-24 Root fracture of maxillary left incisor.

FIG 4-25 The fracture is 4 mm below the gingival margin.

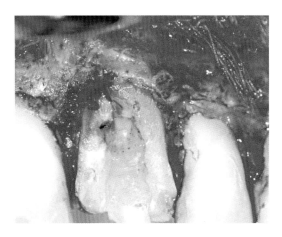
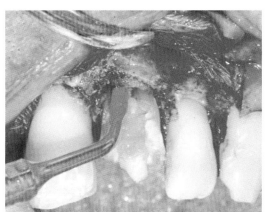

FIG 4-26 The fractured root is ankylotic in the buccal portion.

FIG 4-27 The EX1 insert performs the root resection through the buccal slice technique.

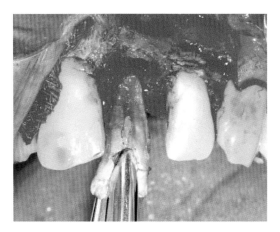
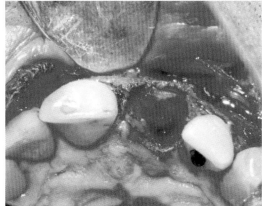

FIG 4-28 The non-ankylotic palatal portion is extracted to create the space necessary to remove the buccal slice.

FIG 4-29 Occlusal view of the ankylotic buccal portion.

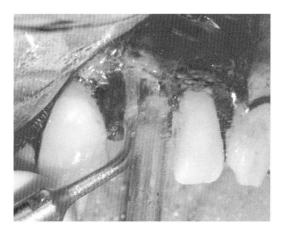

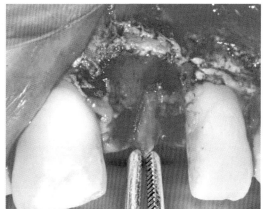

FIG 4-30 Buccal ankylosis removal technique.

FIG 4-31 Buccal fragment removal.

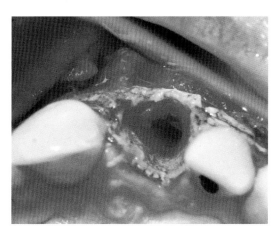

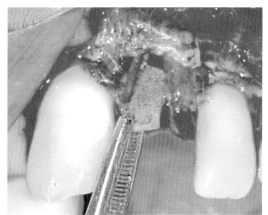

FIG 4-32 Ankylotic buccal portion still attached to the alveolar bone.

FIG 4-33 Last buccal fragment removal.

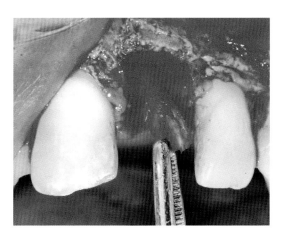

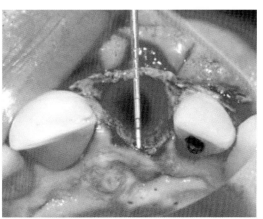

FIG 4-34 Apex removal.

FIG 4-35 Occlusal view showing alveolar integrity following completely ankylotic root extraction on the buccal surface.

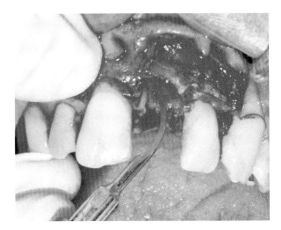
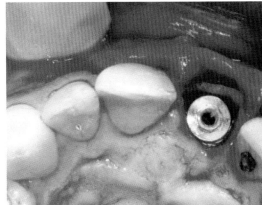

FIG 4-36 The PS2 insert is used to perform alveolar debridement.

FIG 4-37 Implant in position.

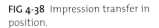
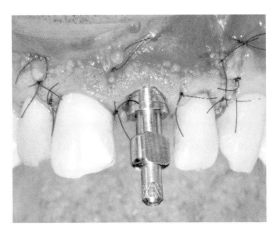
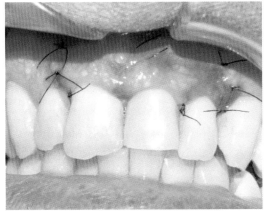

FIG 4-38 Impression transfer in position.

FIG 4-39 Temporary crown placed the day after surgery. The length of the temporary clinical crown was reduced to prevent contact during the parafunction movements (courtesy Dr. Robello).

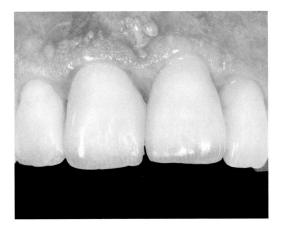
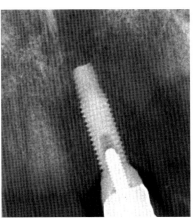

FIG 4-40 Front view of final crown (courtesy Dr. Prando).

FIG 4-41 Post load radiograph (2 years later).

CASE III

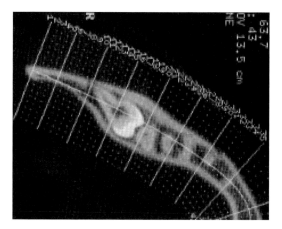
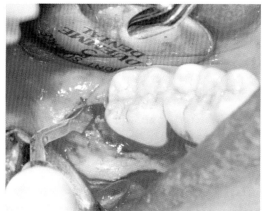

FIG 4-42 CT Sagittal image: notice the dysodontiasis of the third mandibular right molar in the horizontal position.

FIG 4-43 The OP3 insert is used to remove the connective tissue covering the third molar crown at the tip of the crest.

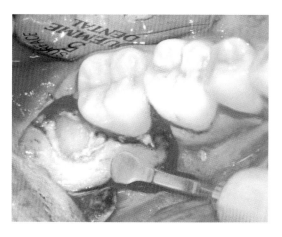
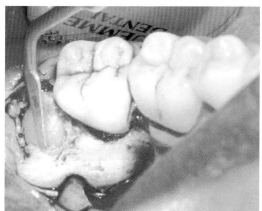

FIG 4-44 The OP3 insert is also used to remove the buccal bone portion and the crown of the impacted tooth is visible.

FIG 4-45 The EX1 insert is used to remove the pericoronal connective tissue.

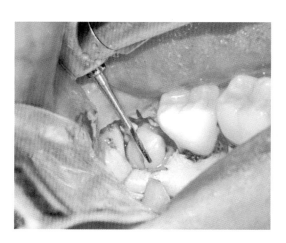
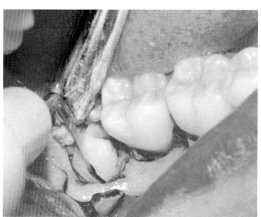

FIG 4-46 A tungsten carbide bur is used to perform a coronal cut in the vestibulo-lingual direction.

FIG 4-47 The EX1 insert is used to finalize the lingual cortical cut.

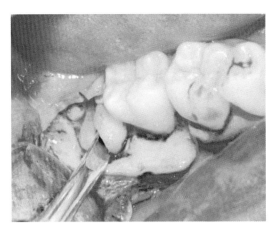

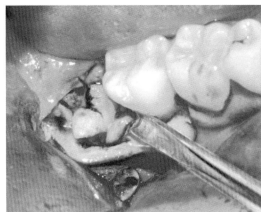

FIG 4-48 A lever is used to fracture the tooth crown.

FIG 4-49 Fractured crown portion.

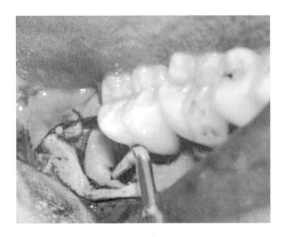

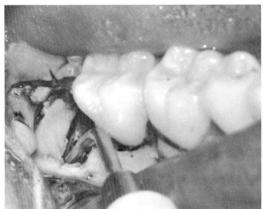

FIG 4-50 The EX1 insert is used to separate the root in the floor of the endodontic space.

FIG 4-51 High intraoperatory visibility thanks to cavitation effect.

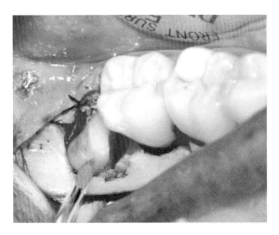

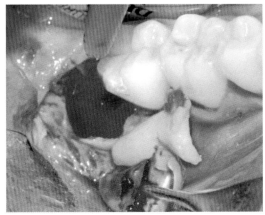

FIG 4-52 A lever is used to remove the distal root.

FIG 4-53 Mesial root removal from deeper position.

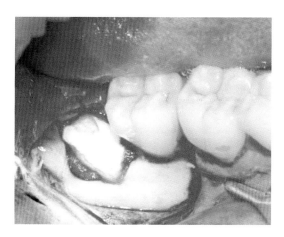 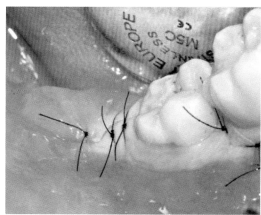

FIG 4-54 After the osteoplasty, the OP3 insert is used to remove surgical alveolar bone fragments where the collagen sponge is placed.

FIG 4-55 Suture.

Crown Lengthening Technique

5

The crown lengthening technique is the most common periodontal resective operation in dentistry.

It is performed for reconstruction when there are cavities that destroy the periodontal surface.

The purpose of lengthening the crown is to place the gingival margin in the apical position. In this way the restoration does not violate the biological spread.

The surgical technique involves lifting the entire flap, pericoronal ostectomy, and making placement more apical to the gingival margin.

This operation is generally limited to posterior sectors because it alters the symmetry of the gingival margin.

The ostectomy technique is the same used in periodontal treatment to restore positive osseous architecture with respect to root emergence.

5.1 Traditional Technique

The traditional technique involves using a bur to perform the ostectomy and restoration osteoplasty.

To prevent accidental contact between the bur and root surface, which might jeopardize the tooth, once the ostectomy and osteoplasty are complete, some bony spikes remain on the root surface and then manual chisels are used.

The bony spikes are removed using manual instruments.

5.2 Surgical Protocol using Piezosurgery

After lifting the primary flap, the secondary flap is removed with the curette-shaped insert (PS 2) for a single tooth or with an OP 3 for a multi-tooth flap.

Scaling is performed with PS 2, whereas debridement of the root surface is performed with OP5.

At this point, the ostectomy is performed while keeping the instrument parallel to the root. In this way, there is no risk of damaging the root.

OP3 can be easily used also in the interproximal region.

Once the ostectomy is complete, smoothing is performed parallel to the root surface and the bony microspikes are removed with the tip of the insert.

Table 5.1 Clinical advantages of using Mectron-Piezosurgery® in periodontal resective surgery

SURGICAL TECHNIQUE	LIMITS OF TRADITIONAL INSTRUMENTS	ADVANTAGES USING PIEZOSURGERY
1. Secondary flap removal	The secondary flap (and also inflamed tissue if there is periodontal illness) is removed using a curette and periodontal chisels. This technique requires great manual skill and there is considerable bleeding.	The secondary flap and inflamed tissue are easily removed using PS2 and OP3. In addition, the saline solution's cavitation effect provides hemostasis and gives maximum visibility.
2. Scaling	Curette and ultrasonic scaler	No difference
3. Ostectomy	The tungsten carbide bur is less traumatic for bony tissue compared to the diamond bur. The bur should never touch the root surface; this is difficult in interproximal spaces when there are natural teeth (not reduced).	The ostectomy with OP3 is more efficient and there is no risk of damaging the root surface. It is used parallel to the surface and does not damage root cement. For interproximal action, OP4 is used, which is an ultrasonic version of the file by Dr. Schlouger.
4. Osteoplasty	The osteoplasty following the ostectomy is to provide a thin osseous profile with respect to root emergence. This technique is highly imprecise and traumatic when using burs, which often pass through the maxillary cortical bone and alter normal osseous morphology. There is a high risk of causing irreversible damage to the root when using the bur in the vicinity. Bone spikes are left to prevent accidental contact with the root. They are then removed with periodontal chisels.	Osteoplasty with Mectron-Piezosurgery® has several advantages. One of the main benefits is that it enables very precise remodeling of the cortical bone without sulci and bleeding even in cases of restoration of tuber maxillae or mandibular tori. A second advantage is that it is possible to gather bone fragments produced during the operation. A third advantage is that it is possible to work in contact with the root. This is why unwanted spikes are not formed as when using the bur.

SURGICAL TECHNIQUE	LIMITS OF TRADITIONAL INSTRUMENTS	ADVANTATES USING PIEZOSURGERY
5. Removal of bony spikes	The bony spikes are removed using manual instruments. This requires difficult and complex searching.	After the ostectomy with OP3 the bony spikes on the root surface are very small and visible only through magnification. They are removed when the root is being smoothened with insert PP1, which ensures a high degree of precision and speed.
6. Bone healing	Bone healing after periodontal surgery has been widely documented in the literature.[1,11,12,23,34,43,52]	Bone healing after crown lengthening using the Mectron-Piezosurgery® technique is more effective from both a clinical and histological standpoint.[74] CLINICAL: light color non-edematous tissue. HISTOLOGICAL: a study was conducted by Harvard University comparing bone healing after crown lengthening using burs and using Mectron-Piezosurgery®. The results showed more favorable bone healing after the osteotomy performed using ultrasound.[67]
7. Root smoothening	Using Gracey curettes provides excellent root smoothening.	Using the PP1 insert enables excellent root smoothening. In only a few seconds, the surface of the cement looks like the surface of enamel.

Dental decay under gingival margin

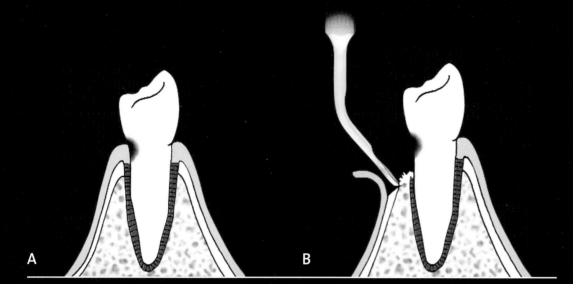

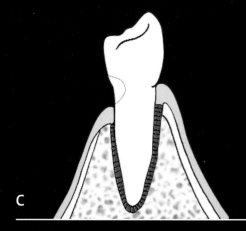

A: Root decay underneath the gingival margin in the lingual view.

B: Ostectomy of the alveolar bone and osteoplasty of the crest bone using the OP3 insert.

C: Tissue healing: the lower edge of the restoration is above the gingival margin thanks to the restoration of the biological mass by placing the lingual flap in an apical direction.

Interproximal cavities

A: Buccal view: interproximal decay in the periodontal tissues at the bone margin.

B: Buccal view: the diamond-coated OP4 insert is placed between the two roots and pressure is applied in apical direction to remove the interproximal bone.

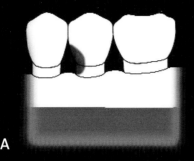

A

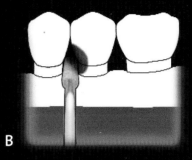

B

C: Lingual view: the insert removes the interproximal bone and cleans the roots.

D: Buccal view: restoration of the biological mass after resective treatment.

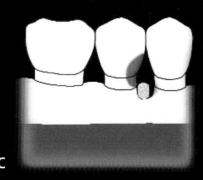

C

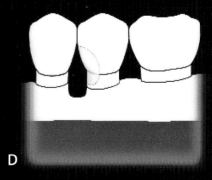

D

CASE I

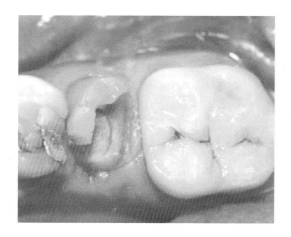

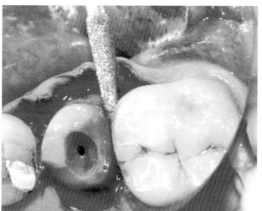

FIG 5-01 Crown fracture of the second mandibular premolar

FIG 5-02 After lifting the entire buccal and lingual flap the OP4 insert is used by applying pressure on the bone crest to perform the interproximal osteotomy and osteoplasty.

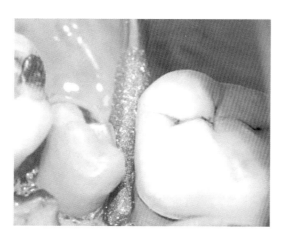

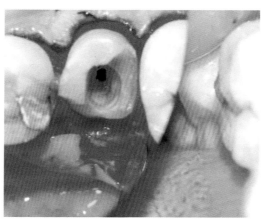

FIG 5-03 Restoring the correct height of the biological mass is made easier by the form of the insert.

FIG 5-04 The OP3 insert is used to perform the lingual and buccal osteotomy and osteoplasty.

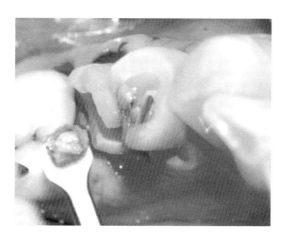

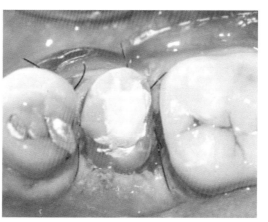

FIG 5-05 Bone fragments collected during the osteoplasty with the OP3 insert.

FIG 5-06 Flap suture with two interrupted stitches.

CASE II

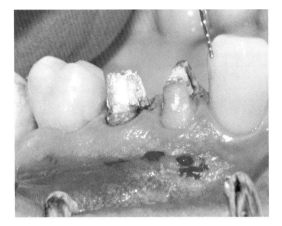
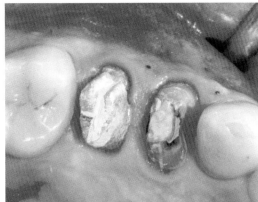

FIG 5-07 Pre-surgery view of the prosthesis stumps with breach of bone mass.

FIG 5-08 Occlusal view.

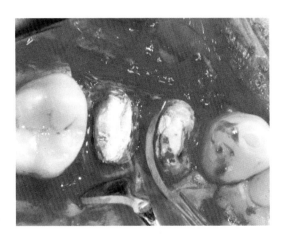
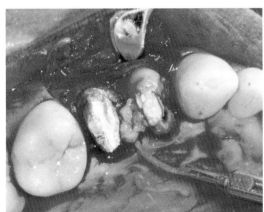

FIG 5-09 and FIG 5-10 Removal of inflamed tissue using the PS2.

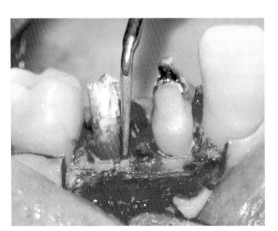
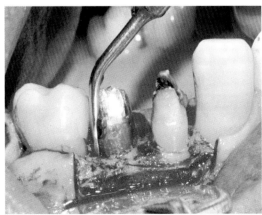

FIG 5-11 Cleaning the root cement using the OP5.

FIG 5-12 Periradicular osteotomy and osteoplasty with the OP3.

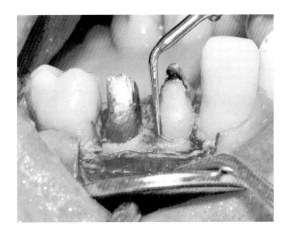

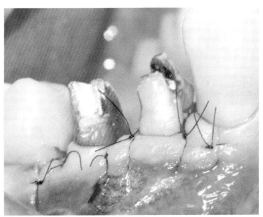

FIG 5-13 Smoothing the root surface and removal of bone spikes using the PP1.

FIG 5-14 Suture with interrupted stitches and placing the flap in apical direction.

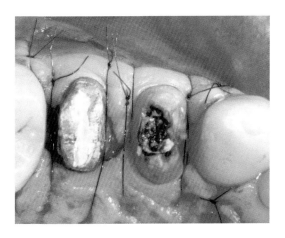

FIG 5-15 Occlusal view.

Ridge Expansion Technique

6

The minimum width of an edentulous crest for placing 4-mm-diameter implants is 6 millimeters in order to obtain at least 1 mm width of buccal and lingual bone side.

Whenever the edentulous site is less than 6 mm in width, it is not possible to place the implant using standard techniques. It is necessary to use an expansion technique or restoration technique.

The technique to follow for each case has to be selected after a careful assessment of the morphology and quality of the edentulous crest, thus detailed presurgery study is necessary.

6.1 Surgical Technique

Horizontal Osteotomy

The horizontal osteotomy is performed on the tip of the edentulous crest. It begins about 1 mm from the periodontium of the last tooth and extends for another 8-10 mm distal to the axis of the last implant desired.

The depth of the cut should be more or less the same length of the implants to be placed.[65]

The bone cut is performed with a 0.55 mm OT7 insert.

Surgeons with experience using Mectron-Piezosurgery® can use a 0.35 mm OT7S insert, which is thinner and more effective.

Vertical Osteotomy

The purpose of the release vertical osteotomy is to enable expansion when the bone is dense. According to the clinical case, the cut is performed at the mesial edge and, where necessary, also the distal edge of the horizontal osteotomy.

It is recommended to extend the release osteotomy as much as possible to prevent fracturing the buccal cortical bone, which, at the apical site, is subject to a joint effect by expansion movement.

This cut must also be a couple og millimeters deep inside the spongy bone.

The insert recommended by the author is OT7S for its width and precision in cutting (illustration 2 on page 60).

Pilot Osteotomy

The pilot osteotomy for each implant site is performed with insert OP5 or IM1. The cone form and microdiamond-coated surface of these inserts makes bone perforation extremely effective and precise also for thin crests. The diameter of the hole made with the inserts is 1.2 mm for OP5 and 2 mm for IM1 (illustration 3).

First Expansion

Expansion screws are immediately inserted in the holes made with OP5 or IM2. The screws have a maximum diameter of 2.5 mm and they expand the buccal cortical space by about 1 mm (illustration 4).

Enlarging the Differential Pilot Osteotomy of the Implant Site

The width of the lingual cortical bone, and if necessary also the buccal cortical bone, is reduced by working inside the pilot osteotomy with the diamond-coated cylinder insert OT4, which is about 2.4 mm in diameter.

This technique developed by the author is termed differential preparation of the implant site.

Differential preparation of the implant site makes it possible to reduce the amount of expansion, especially when there is a 4 to 5 mm bone crest.

Second Expansion

After obtaining the pilot osteotomy of about 3 mm in diameter, a second 3.5 mm expander is inserted, which expands it to a total of only 1.5 mm thanks to the differential preparation.

Placing the Implant

Lastly, a 4-mm-diameter cone implant is placed, which expands it by an additional 0.5 mm.

Once the implant is placed, the final total expansion is about 2 mm, instead of the 4 mm necessary using traditional techniques. This technique makes it possible to achieve minimum invasive surgery and to obtain a normal crest width of 6 mm with about 1 mm of buccal and lingual bone thickness around the implant (illustration 6).

Table 6.1 Clinical advantages of using Mectron-Piezosurgery® in the Ridge Expansion Technique

SURGICAL TECHNIQUE	LIMITS OF TRADITIONAL INSTRUMENTS	ADVANTAGES USING PIEZOSURGERY
1. Osteotomy	The osteotomy technique with bone burs powered by micromotors is traumatic, with little surgical control and is thus not very precise also for the ridge expansion technique. The width of the thinnest bur takes about 1.5 mm and, in addition, there is a limit to depth due to the larger diameter of the bur bit. Vertical osteotomy cannot be performed without damaging the crest bone because it is too traumatic. It is not possible to place the implant at the correct distance in the proximity of the distal periodontium. In conclusion, the characteristics of traditional instruments have limited the use of the ridge expansion technique.	The ultrasonic technique has a minimum degree of invasion. It is precise, quick and guarantees excellent intra-operative control. The width of the osteotomy is 0.60 mm when using insert OT7 and down to 0.40 when using OT7S for vertical cuts. The osteotomy can be as deep as the clinical needs require. Piezoelectric bone surgery developed by the author was presented in the literature for the first time with the publication of a case report on a ridge expansion that was so severe due to its morphology and mineralization that it was not possible to use any other instrument.[64]
2. Pilot osteotomy	The ball bur perforates the cortical bone through considerable pressure on the handle, thereby reducing surgical control when the crest is thin. Thus, it is easy to damage the bone.	The insert OP5 or IM1 is highly precise even when the crest is very thin. It is also efficient and can reach a depth of about 10 mm inside the crest.
3. Differential implant site preparation	Not possible with traditional instruments.	Using the diamond coated insert OT4 makes it possible to extend the pilot osteotomy in order to reduce the amount of expansion millimeters needed. All one needs is 2 mm expansion to place a 4-mm implant in a 4-mm crest. This technique made it possible to speed up tissue healing and to deal with cases where there is a low degree of elasticity due to high density spongy bone.

A: After lifting the flap with mixed thickness (partial in the buccal part and total on the lingual side), a periodontal probe is used to measure the bone crest – 4 mm thick.

B: With the microsaw insert (Mectron-Piezosurgery® OT7), the horizontal osteotomy is performed starting 1 mm distal from the last natural tooth. The buccal corticotomy is performed with Mectron-Piezosurgery® OT7S from the outside or with OP5 from the inside.

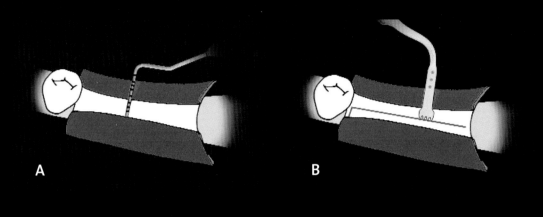

A

B

C: The first holes are made every 7.5 mm using the conical diamond coated Mectron-Piezosurgery® OP5 or IM1.

D: The buccal cortical bone is moved 1 mm from the lingual cortical bone using expander no. 1.

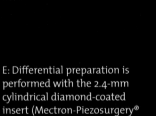
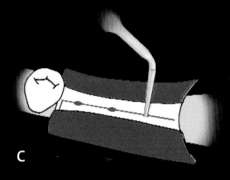
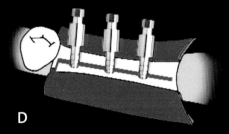

C

D

E: Differential preparation is performed with the 2.4-mm cylindrical diamond-coated insert (Mectron-Piezosurgery® OP4). This manouvre consists of reducing the inside of the lingual cortical bone surface.

F: After placing the implants, about 2 mm of expansion is observed. The expanded bone crest is about 6 mm and the thickness of the buccal/lingual cortical bone is 1 mm.

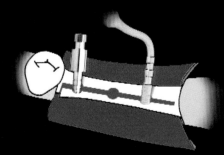
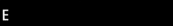
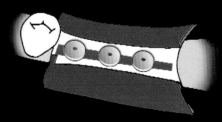

E

F

CASE I

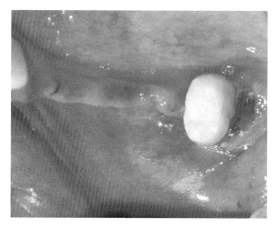
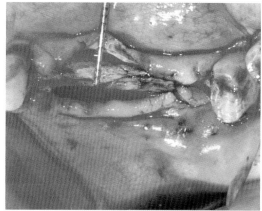

FIG 6-01 Distal edentulous mandible with a natural distal tooth that cannot be recovered but is useful for the temporary bridge during implant integration.

FIG 6-02 The width of the crest is 3 mm after lifing the flap.

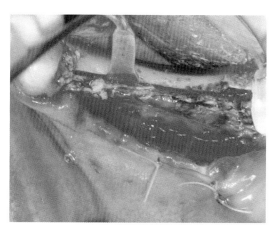
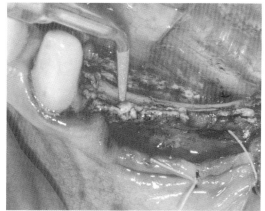

FIG 6-03 Insert OT7 is used to perform a horizontal osteotomy on the tip of the osseous crest. Notice the integrity of the periosteum on the buccal side.

FIG 6-04 Insert OP5 is used to begin preparation of the implant site.

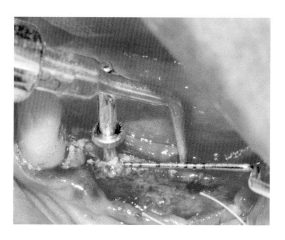
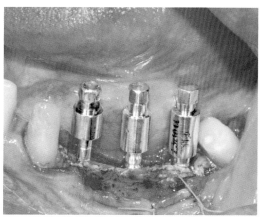

FIG 6-05 The initial pilot osteotomy of the second implant is executed after placing the first pin.

FIG 6-06 Expander no. 1 (2.5 mm max diameter) placed in the initial pilot osteotomies.

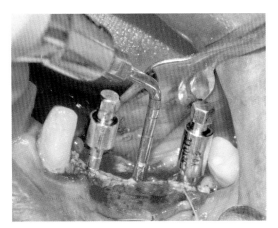

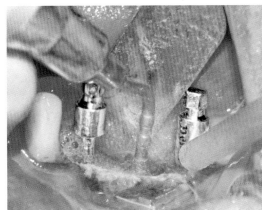

FIG 6-07 Insert IM2 is used after removing expander no. 1.

FIG 6-08 Insert OT4 is used for differential preparation inside the implant site on the lingual cortical crest or bone.

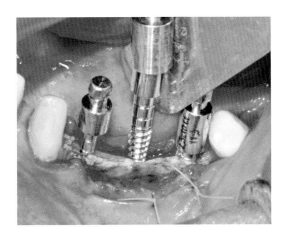

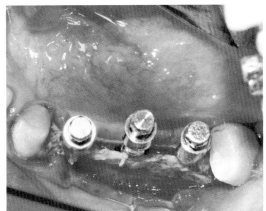

FIG 6-09 Now the 3.5-mm-diameter expander 2 is inserted.

FIG 6-10 Occlusal view of the expansion of the central implant site.

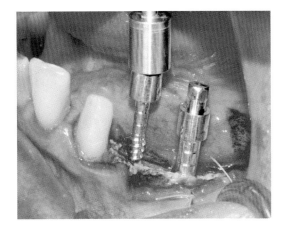

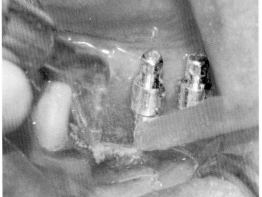

FIG 6-11 The 2.5-mm-diameter expander is removed from the mesial implant site.

FIG 6-12 Differential preparation of the inner lingual cortical bone is executed at the mesial implant site.

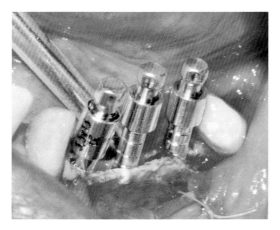

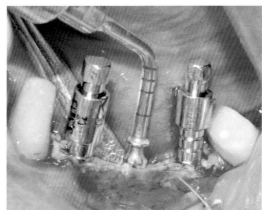

FIG 6-13 Expansion is completed also at the mesial site by placing the 3.5-mm expander.

FIG 6-14 Site preparation is completed with insert IM3.

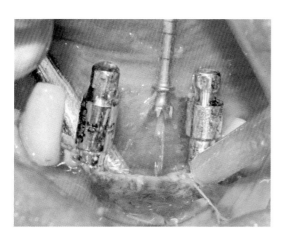

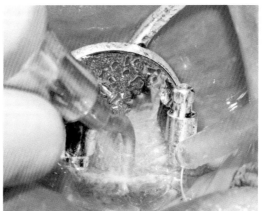

FIG 6-15 Notice the dual irrigation of the insert, which enables removal of spongy bone fragments.

FIG 6-16 Micromechanical vibrations give the cut a porous surface that is perfectly clean thanks to cavitation. In addition, it is thought that ultrasonic waves are able to stimulate cell mitosis.

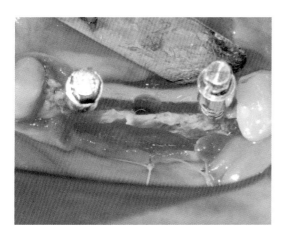

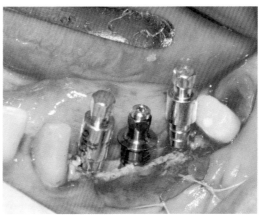

FIG 6-17 Preparation of the implant site complete; notice the crescent on the buccal cortical bone resulting from differential preparation. This makes it possible to reduce the space between the buccal cortical bone (thinner) and the lingual cortical bone (thicker).

FIG 6-18 Insertion of a 4-mm-diameter cone implant ends expansion.

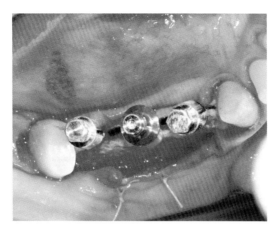
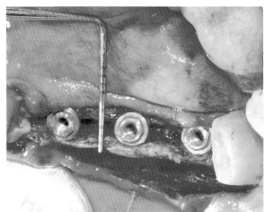

FIG 6-19 Occlusal view of the expansion after placing the median implant.

FIG 6-20 Placement of the three implants completes expansion.

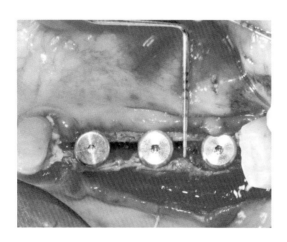
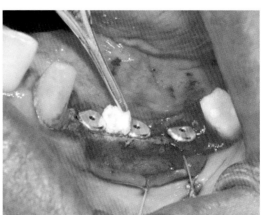

FIG 6-21 Notice how the differential preparation has enabled about 2 mm separation of the two cortical bone.

FIG 6-22 Collagen sponge graft.

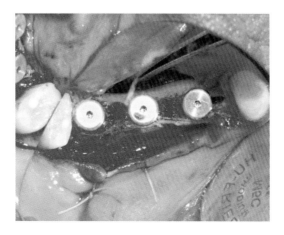
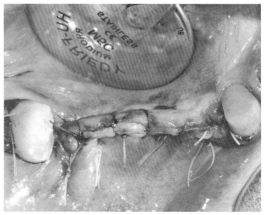

FIG 6-23 Final result: implant in correct prosthesis position (the distal tooth is removed after osseointegration).

FIG 6-24 Suture.

Maxillary Sinus Lift Technique

7

Maxillary sinus surgery for implant purposes enables placement of implants in the posterior maxilla when the crest bone is not sufficiently high.

The access osteotomy that allows lifting the sinus membrane can be performed through a buccal approach or crest approach.

The crest approach, as proposed by Robert Summer, is performed using manual osteotomy and then the vibrations of a hammer are applied. This technique is most effective when there is soft bone. However, when the crest bone is mineralized, using manual instruments is traumatic and not very effective.

In the latter cases, the crest can be prepared and the membrane lifted by using a Mectron-Piezosurgery® diamond-coated insert designed for that purpose. This technique uses ultrasonic microvibrations to ablate the crest bone and uses the cavitation effect of the saline solution to push the bioglass, and then the membrane is lifted.

The author considers this a master technique, because the integrity of the membrane cannot be seen during the operation. Thus, the success of this method mainly depends on the skill and experience of the doctor performing the surgery.

The buccal approach is presented by the author as the only predictable technique because the operator can check that the schneiderian membrane remains intact throughout the operation. In addition, antrostomy of the lateral sinus wall can be performed regardless of any residual anatomy of the alveolar crest. Furthermore, the grafting material is placed only after having checked that the membrane is intact. This makes it possible to prevent complications and failure.

Using Mectron-Piezosurgery®, in the maxillary sinus lift technique with a lateral approach is beneficial throughout the operation.

7.1 Surgical Technique

The surgical technique is divided into five phases.

- **Phase 1: Osteoplasty to thin out the buccal wall of the maxilla**
  With the OP3 osteoplastic insert, the width of buccal bone is reduced until it is possible to see the darker part of the sinus cavity, which indicates the exact position of the sinus cavity. It is recommendable to leave a thin bony wall attached to the membrane. The wall should be about 0.5 mm thick.
  The thinning action simultaneously produces bone fragments that can be used later as grafting material.

- **Phase 2: Bony window osteotomy**
  Once the bone wall reaches a width of less than one millimeter, bony window osteotomy is performed through a cutting action with an OT1 diamond-coated scalpel in order to trace the frame of the bony window.
  The ideal form of the window is oval, in order to follow the length of the sinus floor and to make the operation faster. In this way, the characteristic angles of a rectangular window are not formed.
  The dimensions of the bony window are generally about 5 or 6 mm in height while the length depends on the number of implants planned.

The cut is made with the vertical portion of the OT1 diamond-coated insert.
In this way, the width of the bone is removed where the color of the sinus membrane appears, which is the frame of the window.
The correct technique entails a clear cut and not a consumption of the bone.

- **Phase 3: Separation of the sinus membrane**
  Separation of the sinus membrane, conceived by the author, is aimed at eliminating membrane tension to ease lifting. A special insert is used (EL1) in the shape of an inverted blunt cone, which separates the membrane itself by about 2 mm, by running it along the inside perimeter of the bony window.

- **Phase 4: Lifting the sinus membrane**
  After phase 3, once membrane mobility is reached, the author generally performs the lift using manual lifters with sharp ends. Using Mectron-Piezosurgery® inserts EL2, EL3 and OP3 facilitates lifting when the membrane is attached to the floor.

- **Phase 5: Preparation of implant site**
  Preparation of the implant site using Mectron-Piezosurgery® is possible even when there is a very thin residual crest. The inserts used are those in the implant kit (IM1, IM2, OT4, IM3).

Table 7.1 Clinical advantages of using Mectron-Piezosurgery® in the maxillary sinus lift technique

SURGICAL TECHNIQUE	LIMITS OF TRADITIONAL INSTRUMENTS	ADVANTAGES USING PIEZOSURGERY
1. Osteoplasty technique and collecting bone fragments	Not possible	Thinning osteoplasty offers two important clinical benefits. The first depends on a reduction of the bone wall, which makes it possible to precisely localize the sinus cavity, which is darker than the crest bone. The second advantage is the ability to gather bone fragments to add to the grafting material.
2. Bony window osteotomy technique ***	The bur reaches the membrane while consuming bone. If the bur accidentally touches the membrane it is easily perforated. In the literature, the average perforation rate is 30% when using burs.	The Mectron-Piezosurgery® diamond-coated insert, which is characterized by its selective cut, makes a net cut along the entire width, without perforating the membrane on contact. In the literature, the average perforation rate using Mectron-Piezosurgery® is 7%. This rate also includes the learning curve.[65,80] In addition, the dimensions and form of the bony window are optimal with respect to sinus anatomy.
3. Separation of the sinus membrane	There are no instruments that perform this function.	By applying a special insert in the shape of an inverted blunt cone, it is possible to separate the membrane around the perimeter of the bony window. This separation eliminates any membrane tension, which becomes loose and makes it easier to use manual instruments for subsequent lifting.[74,75]

SURGICAL TECHNIQUE	LIMITS OF TRADITIONAL INSTRUMENTS	ADVANTAGES USING PIEZOSURGERY
4. Preparation of implant site	With twist drills, it is possible to prepare the implant site when the residual crest is at least 4 mm high and adequately thick. If it is less, then it is difficult to obtain sufficient initial implant stability and it is possible to fracture the bone crest.	Preparation of the implant site with Mectron-Piezosurgery®, based on microvibrations, makes it possible to better exploit any residual anatomy, thus preventing crest fractures and making it possible to obtain sufficient initial stability even when there are only 2 or 3 mm of residual crest. This characteristic is extremely important because it makes it possible to solve the majority of critical atrophy in the maxilla in only one surgical operation.

*** The literature reveals how osteotomy of the maxillary lateral wall for sinus surgery performed with burs results in perforating the Schneiderian membrane in 14% to 15% of cases, depending on the operator.[8,58,59,80]
Using Mectron Piezosurgery®, this percentage is reduced considerably, to a percentage that varies from 0 to 23% of cases according to the skill of the operator.[2]
In a recent article published by New York University, the authors demonstrated how the percentage of perforation in 100 consecutive cases using Mectron Piezosurgery® drops to 7%, compared to 30% obtained, by the same operators, using burs.[80]

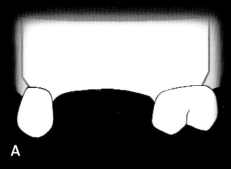

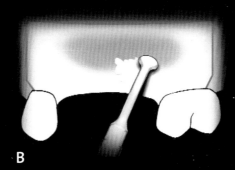

A: Full thickness flap raised. Lateral bony sinus wall in white color.

B: Thinning osteoplasty: the OP3 insert is used to reduce thickness of the lateral sinus wall until the dark color indicating the sinus cavity is visible.

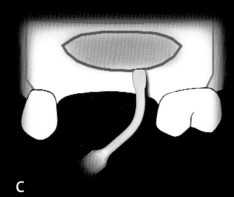

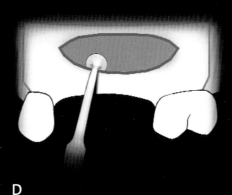

C: Access Osteotomy: the OT1 diamond-coated insert is used to outline bony window contour. Consequently, bony window osteotomy is performed applying a traction motion to the insert's vertical part. The Schneiderian membrane exposure corresponds to the red color of the bony window. An oval shape is considered ideal. The bony window is then cautiously detached from the Schneiderian membrane.

D: Membrane separation: the EL1 insert is used along the inner perimeter of the bony window to separate the sinus membrane by about 2 mm towards the outside.

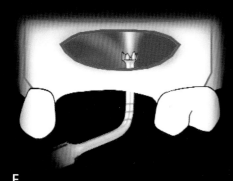

E: After manually elevating the Schneiderian membrane and protecting it with collagen membrane and sponges, the implant site is prepared using the proper inserts (IM1-IM2-OT4-IM3). Correct implant site preparation using Piezosurgery enables sufficient primary stability even when the residual crest is only 2-3 mm.

CASE I

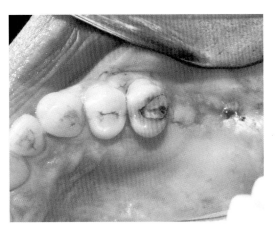
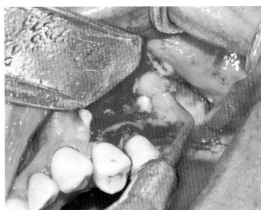

FIG 7-01 Maxillary left molars missing.

FIG 7-02 Osteoplasty performed with the OP3 insert reduces the thickness of the lateral maxillary sinus wall to less than 1 mm. The bone fragments harvested will then be used for grafting.

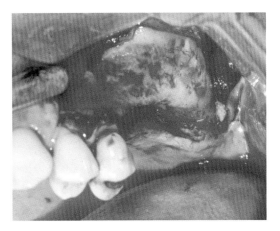
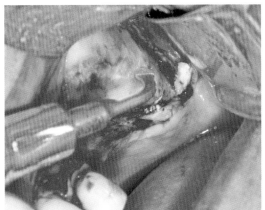

FIG 7-03 When the osteoplasty is completed, the dark color of the sinus cavity will be clearly visible, due to the contrast with the light color of the notably reduced residual crestal bone.

FIG 7-04 Cutting action is initiated by using the inner edge of the OT1 insert.

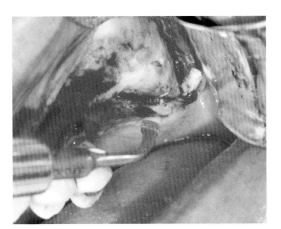
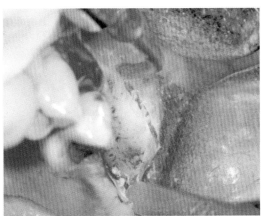

FIG 7-05 Initial osteotomy.

FIG 7-06 OT1 cuts through the bony wall thickness.

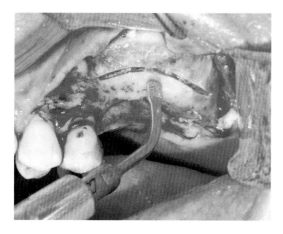

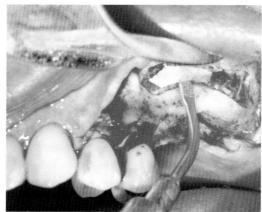

FIG 7-07 The osteotomy performed with the OT1 insert defines an osseous frame which reflects sinus floor anatomy.

FIG 7-08 The bony window is removed following completion of the osteotomy.

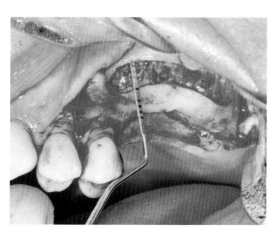

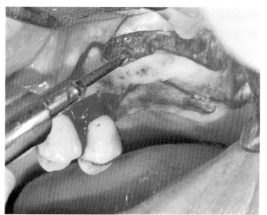

FIG 7-09 Ideally, the completed bony window should be approximately 5 mm high and as long as possible in respect to the position of the implants.

FIG 7-10 The EL1 insert is used to start separation of the membrane, which is detached for 2 mm along the bony window frame.

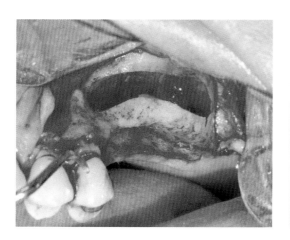

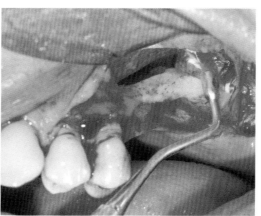

FIG 7-11 The Scheneiderian membrane is lifted with a manual elevator

FIG 7-12 Collagen sponges are grafted into the distal part of the sinus to reduce bone graft size in areas where implants will not be set.

FIG 7-13 A conical diamond-coated insert (OP5/IM1) is used to begin implant site preparation.

FIG 7-14 Inserts IM1 or IM2 are used to perform pilot osteotomy.

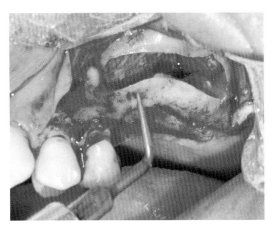

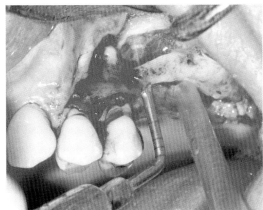

FIG 7-15 The OP4 insert is used to perform differential preparation to optimize implant axis.

FIG 7-16 Experienced surgeons can obtain primary stability even when residual crest width is only 1 mm.

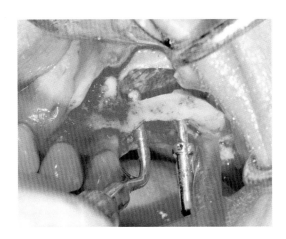

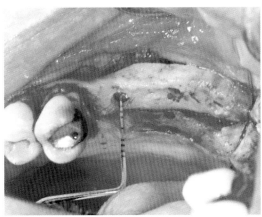

FIG 7-17 The IM3 insert is used for final site preparation.

FIG 7-18 Occlusal view of implant site preparation.

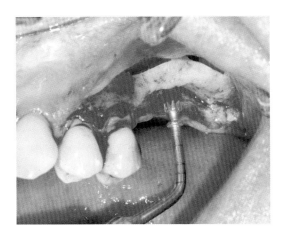

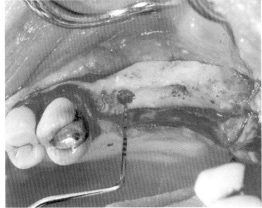

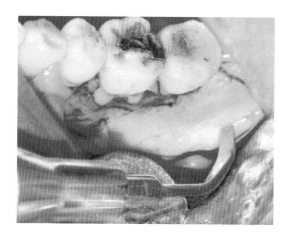

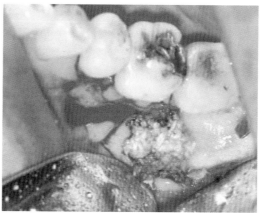

FIG 7-19 Donor site in the mandibular molar region: the OP1.

FIG 7-20 Bone chips are harvested by setting irrigation at the lowest level and keeping suction in the opposite direction of collection.

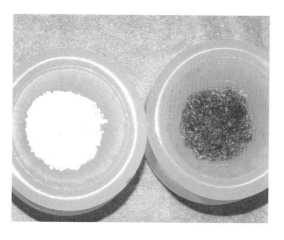

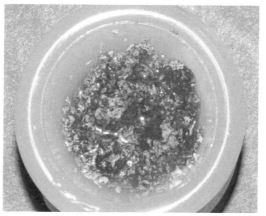

FIG 7-21 Bone chips are collected in a container and are later mixed with bovine hydroxyapatite.

FIG 7-22 The graft composite has a volume of 2.5 cc.

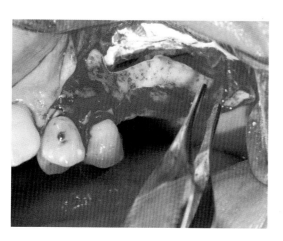

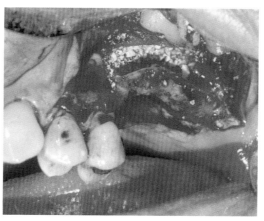

FIG 7-23 A resorbable membrane is inserted to cover the schneiderian membrane.

FIG 7-24 The resorbable membrane protects the sinus membrane from bovine hydroxyapatite coarseness.

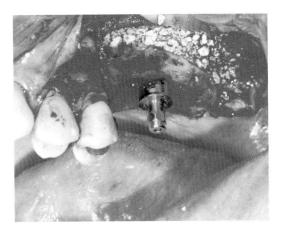

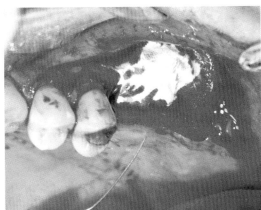

FIG 7-25 Implant positioning.

FIG 7-26 The bony window is covered with collagen membrane.

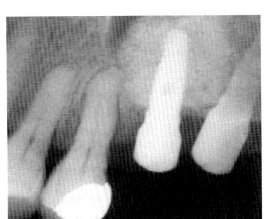

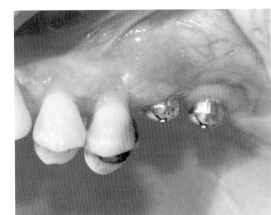

FIG 7-27 Radiograph at time of reopening (6 months later).

FIG 7-28 Gingival healing following buccal placement.

Bone Grafting Techniques

8

Intra-oral bone harvesting in monocortical blocks is a technique that is increasingly being used to correct defects in the edentulous crest which have to be restored with dental implants.

The donor site is selected based on the size of the defect and based on the amount of bone available in the mandible and/or maxillary bone.

The anatomic region used most frequently for bone harvesting is the ramus and body of the mandible, since in most cases, they provide enough bone to correct a ridge defect of two or three elements. This area also carries very limited anatomical risk.

Another donor site, even if not prime, is the chin symphysis in the event of thick bucco-lingual and limited root length of front teeth. This anatomical region is easily accessible with surgery, but it requires opening a broad mucogingival flap to prevent neurological consequences that may follow the technique, which entails direct incision in the buccal fornix.

Generally, if little bone is needed, it can be harvested from the mandibular tori or the area of the tuber maxillae.

The choice to perform block osseous graft or restoration techniques using particulate bone is made preoperatively, after carefully examining the anatomy of the defect and tissue properties.

The bone graft is successful only if it is performed by closely following the surgical protocol, both for soft and mineralized tissue.

This chapter illustrates only a few surgical aspects and clinical benefits of harvesting a monocortical block from the mandible and placement in the receiving site to correct a defect in the thickness of the edentulous crest.

8.1 Surgical Technique

Preparing the Receiving Site

The reduced thickness of the bucco-lingual osseous crest produces a defect in the edentulous ridge characterized by a concavity with respect to the emergence of adjacent natural teeth (fig. A, page 80).

Measuring the Ridge Defect

It is necessary to measure the thickness of the crest to determine the severity of the defect. This assessment is possible only in the central region of the concavity and it in itself does not enable assessment of the size of the defect and does not provide useful indications on the morphology necessary to determine the bone withdrawn.

Morphology of the Ridge Defect

The author proposes a preliminary remodeling technique to modify the bone defect until the site is geometrically more favorable for measurement and subsequent application of the monocortical graft block. This osteoplasty is performed with an insert for that purpose (OP1), which is square-shaped and sharp on all sides. The OP1 insert works on the defect on the edges of the concavity in order to obtain flat surfaces that meet at angles (fig. B, page 80).

The linear surfaces thus obtained can be measured with precision using a millimeter probe.

Measurement of the parallelepiped sides obtained makes it possible to determine the exact morphology of the block needed (fig. C, page 81).

The remodeling action produces bone fragments that are collected and used later as grafting material between the receiving site and osseous block.

This osseous micrograft, according to the author, enables homeostasis and tissue healing, thus favoring postoperative recovery. Homeostasis and tissue healing are thought to be due to exposure to a high number of BMP (bio-morphogenetic proteins) following ultrasonic micronization of the cortical bone.

Harvesting from the Mandibular Ramus and Body

Once the dimensions and morphology of the bone graft are determined, the bone is harvested from the donor site.

Selecting the harvest area in the posterior section of the mandible depends on the amount of bone available in the mandibular body and ramus (fig. D, page 81).

To help assess the amount to harvest, it is important to assess the characteristics and dimensions of the external oblique line in the molar region.

By applying the measurements taken at the receiving site with a periodontal probe, the best area for the donor site is determined.

The bone surgery technique consists of performing a horizontal osteotomy medially to the external oblique line until the thickness desired is obtained. The width of the OT7 insert should be taken into consideration, which is 0.55 mm (*).

The OT7 insert has notches on the blade that help perform the osteotomy for the entire length necessary. Again with the OT7, the two horizontal osteotomies are performed until meeting the horizontal cut just made (fig. E, page 80).

The base osteotomy is performed with special inserts, at angles on the left and right sides (OT8 L or R), which prevent damage to the deeper part of the flap (fig. F, page 80).

The author stresses that every osteotomy should reach and surpass the cross-point with the others.

In this way, once piezoelectric surgery is complete, the monocortical block can be removed easily without using a chisel.

This fact is very important from a clinical standpoint, because it is possible only after cutting the internal surface, so that at the end, the thickness of the spongy bone is uniform.

Technique to Prepare the Block Removed

Using an osteoplasty insert (OP1 or OP3), the operator holds the material between his/her fingers and models it to adapt it to the morphology of the receiving site.

With insert OP5, the two holes are made to place the screws (fig. G, page 81).

Technique for Placing the Bone Graft in the Receiving Site

After placing the graft in the receiving site, it is kept in place using fingers or special forceps. The residual bone crest is reached in depth using insert OP5 through the hole already present in the block.

The screws are placed immediately and should be stable in the receiving site, but passive when passing through the block where the hole is slightly wider (fig. H, page 81). This prevents the graft from being dislocated when the screws are tightened.

Insert the first screw, and once the graft is stable, it is easy to place the second.

Once the block is secure, a restoration osteoplasty is performed with insert OP3 to eliminate any sharp corners.

(*) Surgeons who are experienced in using Mectron-Piezosurgery® can perform the osteotomy with a thinner insert, which is much faster and more precise. The OT7S insert is only 0.35 mm in width and should be used by setting the power on the device to Special.

Table 8.1 : Clinical advantages of using Mectron-Piezosurgery® in the bone grafting techniques

SURGICAL TECHNIQUE	LIMITS OF TRADITIONAL INSTRUMENTS	ADVANTAGES USING PIEZOSURGERY
1. Preparation of receiving site	Burs and chisels require difficult and complex inquiry and prevent gathering bone fragments.	Quick and precise while collecting bone fragments.
2. Technique to withdraw the monocortical block	The osteotomy technique with bone burs powered by micromotors is traumatic, very slow and with little surgical control. The horizontal osteotomy is performed by producing several holes, in the width of the cortical bone, which are then connected to each other. Considering the fact that the thinnest burs have a diameter of about 1 mm, the cut produced by macrovibrations entails losing about 1.5 mm in graft width. In addition, for this reason, the cutting action is limited to the width of the cortical bone. As a consequence, the cut of the internal spongy surface is not even because it is torn after dislocating the block with a chisel. This results in an irregular internal surface of the block. The thickness of spongy bone is irregular and so it has to be remodeled in order to place it in the receiving site, which means additional thickness is lost.	Quick and precise technique with maximum intra-operatory control and visibility. The width of the osteotomy is 0.60 mm when using insert OT7, and down to 0.40 when using OT7S. It is possible to perform a deep cut on the internal surface of the graft. In this way, spongy bone has a flat surface. Harvesting with piezosurgery enables osseous tissue to be conserved. The author usually collects bone fragments near the donor site to use them later as grafting material between the receiving site and osseous block. An additional clinical benefit is the very fast postoperative recovery rate compared to the bur. Harvesting time is much more precise and quick compared to the bur.
3. Technique to prepare the block	Requires difficult and complex inquiry with loss of restored osseous particles. The holes for the screws have to be made prior to removing the block from the donor site due to bur rotation.	The operator very quickly performs the restoration osteoplasty and makes holes for the screws while holding the block between his/her fingers.

SURGICAL TECHNIQUE	LIMITS OF TRADITIONAL INSTRUMENTS	ADVANTAGES USING PIEZOSURGERY
4. Grafting technique for the receiving site	Preparation of the holes in the residual crest can require difficult and complex inquiry because bur rotation tends to dislocate the graft.	Preparation of the holes in the residual crest is extremely precise, very safe and saves time.
5. Graft remodeling	Very imprecise with loss of bone fragments.	Very accurate and bone fragments are immediately grafted to fill the spaces between the graft and receiving site.[50]

A: The bone defect is generally a concave that is difficult to measure

B: OP1 is used to deepen the defect until the walls are flat

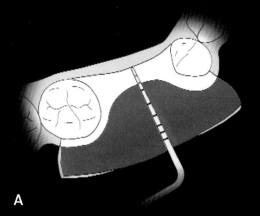

A

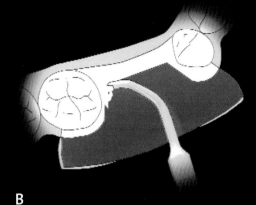

B

E: Insert OT7 is used to perform the horizontal osteotomy incision to the external oblique line and to the depth required. The two vertical incisions are performed with the same insert

F: Insert OT8 is used to perform the horizontal osteotomy incision at the apex until reaching the horizontal incision made with the OT7

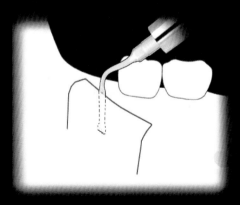

E

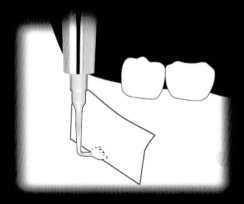

F

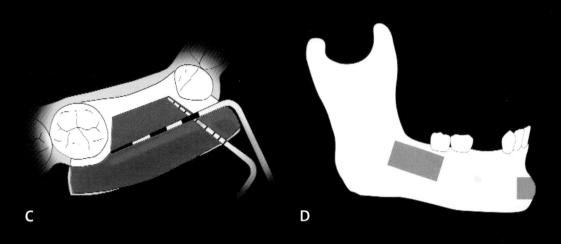

C

D

C: A periodontal probe is used to obtain a precise measurement of the bone defect

D: The red rectangles mark the ideal position of the donor site for harvesting the monocortical block. The rectangle in the back area corresponds to the ramus and body of the mandible near the external oblique line. At chin level the rectangle is placed 4-5 mm apically with respect to the natural tooth apexes

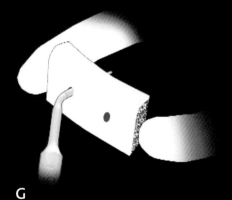

G

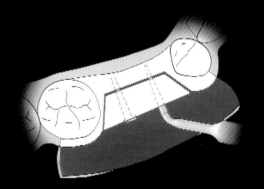

H

G: OP5 is used to make the holes at about 5 mm from the mesial and distal ends while holding the bone graft in your fingers

H: While keeping the insert in position you cross the graft with OP5 to make the screw hole in the receiving site

CASE I

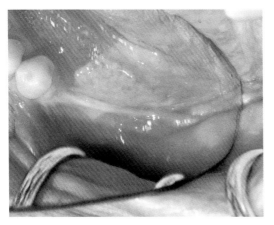
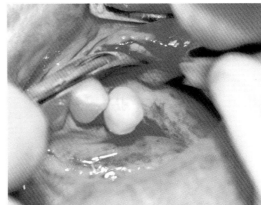

FIG 8-01 Distal edentulous region at first mandibular premolar with critical crest absorption and loss of gingiva.

FIG 8-02 Exposure of tooth nerve emergence.

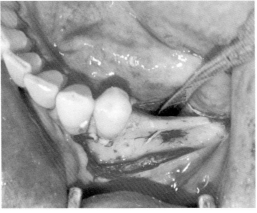
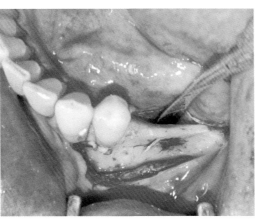
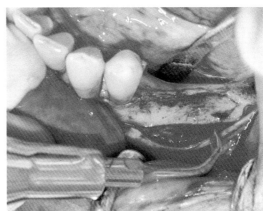

FIG 8-03 The bone morphology is assessed from the lingual view.

FIG 8-04 Insert OP1 is used to prepare the surface of the receiving site.

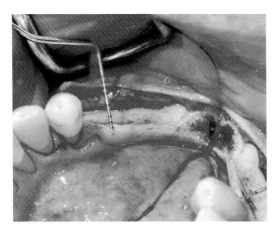
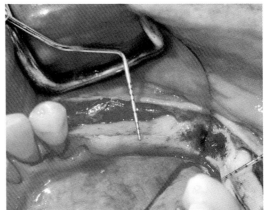

FIG 8-05 The crest width is only 2 mm at the position of the first implant.

FIG 8-06 The crest width is only 1 mm at the position of the second implant.

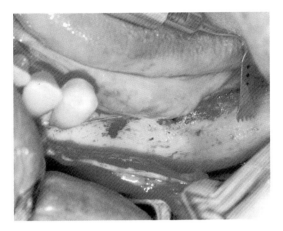

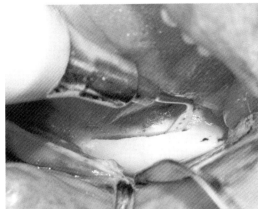

FIG 8-07 The external oblique line is assessed to determine the harvest area.

FIG 8-08 Insert OT7 is used to perform the horizontal osteotomy for the entire height necessary.

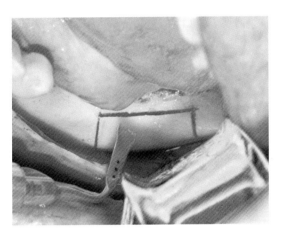

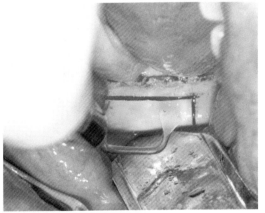

FIG 8-09 The two incisions perpendicular to the horizontal osteotomy are made.

FIG 8-10 Insert OT8 is used to perform the base osteotomy near the angle of the mandible.

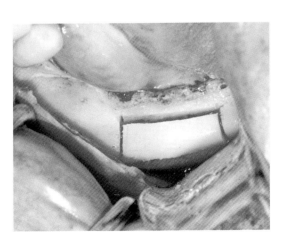

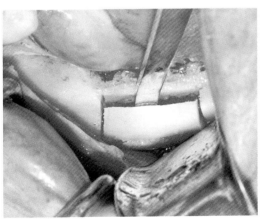

FIG 8-11 The osteotomies are complete.

FIG 8-12 The block is removed.

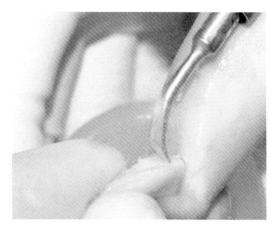
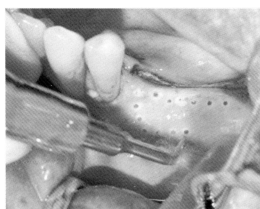

FIG 8-13 The block is remodeled by holding it in one's fingers.

FIG 8-14 Insert OP5 is used to stimulate the bone through buccal surface corticotomies.

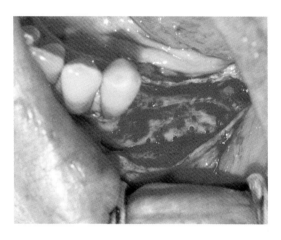
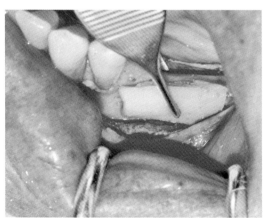

FIG 8-15 Preparation of the vascular bed is complete.

FIG 8-16 The block is checked in the receiving site.

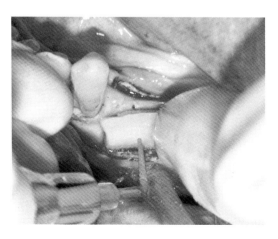
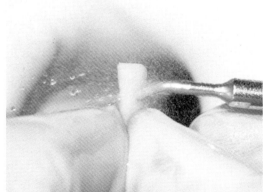

FIG 8-17 Insert OP5 is used to mark the position of the hole for placing the screw.

FIG 8-18 The block hole ends in an extra-oral position.

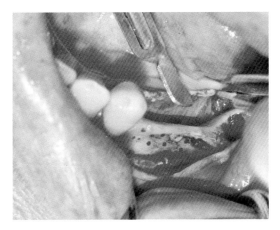

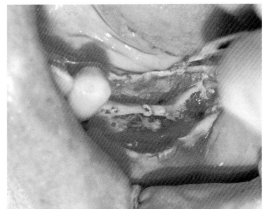

FIG 8-19 The lingual periosteal incision is made with a no. 15 scalpel blade.

FIG 8-20 The lingual flap is lengthened after the incision.

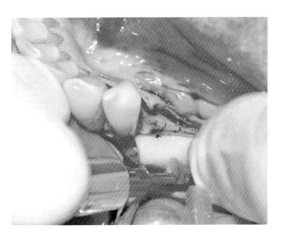

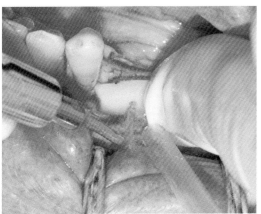

FIG 8-21 Insert OP5 is used to prepare the hole for placing the screw in the receiving site.

FIG 8-22 Insert OT5 is used for screw-head countersink.

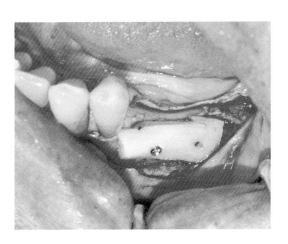

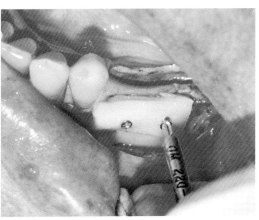

FIG 8-23 The block is fixed with the first screw.

FIG 8-24 The second screw is set after preparing the hole in the receiving site with insert OP5.

FIG 8-25 Insert OP3 is used to perform an osteoplasty to remove sharp edges.

FIG 8-26 The bone graft is in position and the collagen at the donor site is visible.

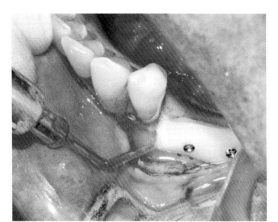
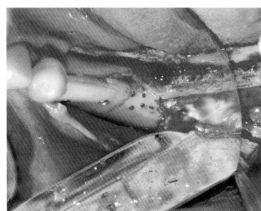

FIG 8-27 OP3 is used to gather bone fragments to place around the graft.

FIG 8-28 A bio-guide membrane is inserted in the lingual flap.

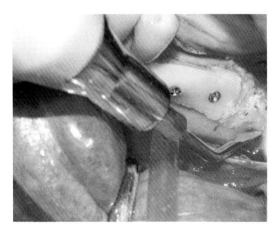
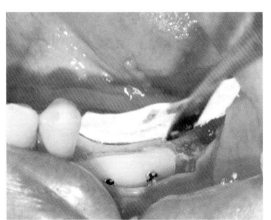

FIG 8-29 Graft in position.

FIG 8-30 Absorbable hydroxyapatite graft (c-graft).

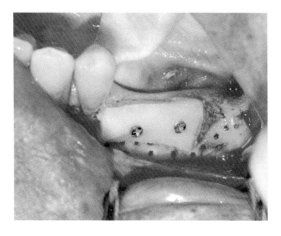
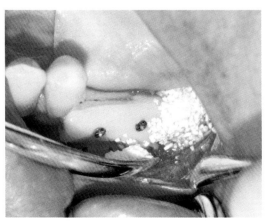

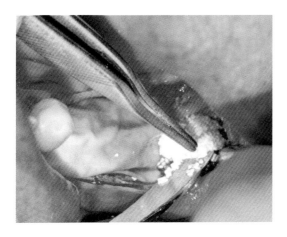

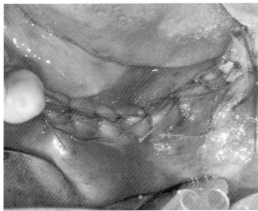

FIG 8-31 Collagen membrane cover and removal of excess hydroxyapatite.

FIG 8-32 Mattress suture and interrupted stitches.

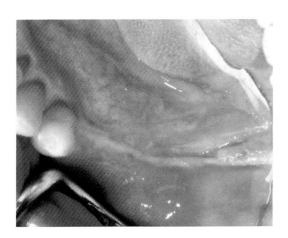

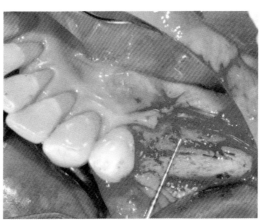

FIG 8-33 Second surgical phase 5 months after graft.

FIG 8-34 Occlusal view of the edentulous crest width with graft in position.

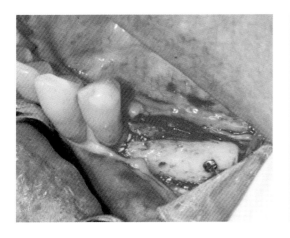

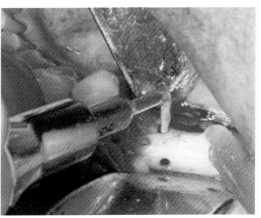

FIG 8-35 Removal of screws.

FIG 8-36 Preparation of the implant site using insert OP5.

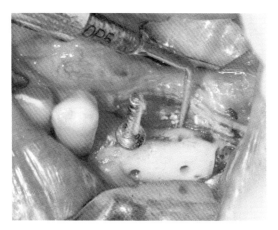 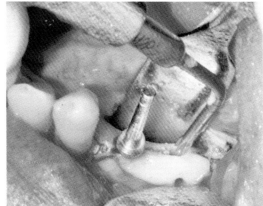

FIG 8-37 Preparation of the implant site and first parallel pin.

FIG 8-38 Preparation of the pilot osteotomy using insert IM2.

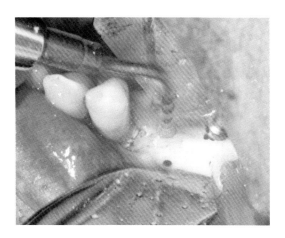 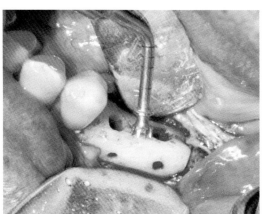

FIG 8-39 Differential preparation technique with insert OT4 to optimize the pilot osteotomy.

FIG 8-40 Final preparation with insert IM3.

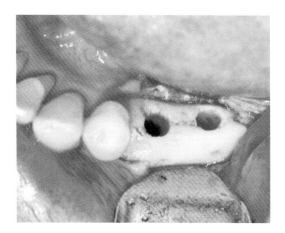 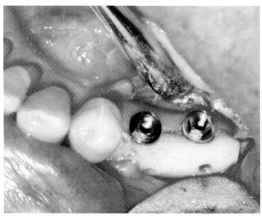

FIG 8-41 Implant sites prepared.

FIG 8-42 Implants in position.

SECTION IV

NEW CONCEPTS AND
NEW SURGICAL TECHNIQUES
USING PIEZOSURGERY

New Bone Classification for Analysis of the Single Surgical Site

Surgical Site Specific Bone Quantity and Quality Classification

Tomaso Vercellotti & Giuseppe Vercellotti
2007

The new bone classification conceived and proposed by the authors Tomaso and Giuseppe Vercellotti has universal application and can be used in all fields of bone surgery, from orthodontics to orthopedics.

In particular, it enables highly precise and simple definition of the anatomy of each surgical site thanks to its dual application for quantitative classification of cortical thickness and qualitative classification of density of spongy bone.

Preoperative analysis based on this classification makes it possible to choose the best cutting instruments and fixation systems for all anatomical areas.

9.1 Application in Implantology

In implantology, preoperative analysis of the bone crest is performed by assessing the paraxial images from computerized tomog-raphy. The classification outlines the quantitative characteristics of the cortical crest and, separately, the density of spongy bone mineralization.

Quantitative Classification

This classification measures the thickness of the Cortical crest, in millimeters.

- **0 mm:** thickness of the cortical crest at the site of recent tooth extraction after a few months.
- **1 mm:** thickness of the cortical crest at the site of tooth extraction after several months.
- **2 mm:** thickness of the cortical crest at the site of tooth extraction after a few years.
- **3 mm o più:** thickness of the cortical crest at the site of tooth extraction after several years and characterized by a reduction in spongy bone resulting in partial merging of the buccal cortical and lingual cortical bone.

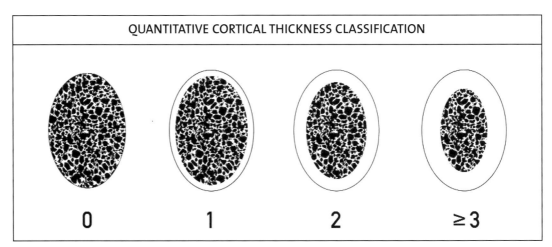

FIG 9-1 Cortical crestal bone. Measurement in mm.

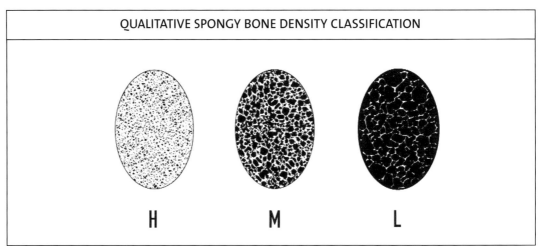

FIG 9-2 Radiopacity vs radiolucency – spongy bone (high – medium - low).

Qualitative Classification Clinically
This classification defines the Density of Spongy Bone.

Spongy bone density is assessed based on the radiotransparency or radio-opacity of the tomographic images.

- **HIGH Density**, to indicate high density of spongy bone. The tomographic image is prevalently radiopaque and grayish-whitish in color.

- **MEDIUM Density**, to indicate medium density of spongy bone. The tomographic image is rather radiopaque and grayish in color.

- **LOW Density**, to indicate low density of spongy bone. The tomographic image is radiolucent and grayish-blackish in color.

Using the Hounsfield unit together with this new classification enables higher precision in defining the degree of spongy bone mineralization and adds a numeric figure to the category identified as H, M, L.

Certainty of Diagnoses

This new classification, which assesses separately and then jointly the characteristics of the cortical and spongy bone, enables certainty of diagnosis by describing every type of tomographic image of the bone anatomy under examination by the surgeon.

Bone Classification and Surgical Decision Making

The classification simplifies surgical decision making.

Indeed, knowing cortical thickness in relation to the degree of spongy bone mineralization helps choose the best instruments to perforate the bone and the best fixation systems.

In dental implantology, it makes it possible to better exploit the anatomical characteristics of each implant site and ensure the highest degree of primary stability possible.

Vercellotti's bone classification also makes it possible to use concepts of bone microsurgery in implantology and, in particular, the new technique of differential preparation of the implant site.

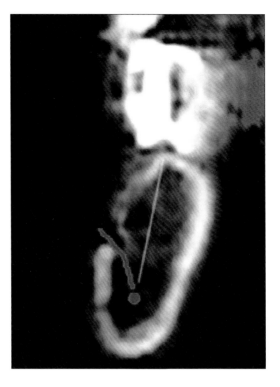

FIG 9-3 Example of pre-implant analysis carried out using the new bone classification system by T&G Vercellotti on a CT image.
Diagnosis:
Cortical crest width 0 mm, density of spongy bone LOW. Surgical decision: Implant site with insufficient anatomical characteristics to obtain acceptable primary stability. This site is not suitable for immediate load.
From a surgical standpoint, the diameter of the implant site should be limited to the pilot osteotomy diameter.

9.2 Conclusions

From a study conducted by the University of Turin, it is clear that using the new bone classification proposed by Tomaso and Giuseppe Vercellotti enables higher precision in preoperative anatomical analysis compared to previous classification systems.

Knowing the characteristics of cortical thickness and density of spongy bone allows the surgeon to choose the best instruments, surgical technique, and implant characteristics, not only to optimize primary stability but also to favor bone healing, which is what determines secondary stability.

The new bone classification is indispensable for correct use of the Ultrasonic Implant Site Preparation Technique and Differential Implant Site Preparation Technique proposed by the author using Mectron-Piezosurgery®.

New Technique of Ultrasonic Implant Site Preparation

10

Over the last ten years, the development of clinical implantology has been steered by the development of implant surface characteristics, which have gone from smooth to ridged, in order to improve bone healing response.

Five years ago, the author decided to study possible development in implantology, focusing his attention on surgical preparation of the implant site.

This research immediately revealed that the technique presented by P.I. Brånemark had not undergone any major developments over the years. Encouraged by the clinical and histological results from using Mectron-Piezosurgery® for osteotomy, he spurred Mectron to develop specific inserts for bone perforation. This was a major technological challenge, because it had never been attempted by anyone else in the past.

Here, published for the first time, is the surgical protocol, instructions and related clinical benefits.

10.1 Surgical Protocol

The surgical protocol entails using inserts whose diameter progressively rises up to 3 mm for a 4-mm implant and 4 mm for a 5-mm implant.

Sequence of inserts:

- IM1 (implant no. 1): the first terminal is a diamond-coated cone insert with a maximum diameter of 2 mm. It replaces the ball bur and is used to begin perforation not only of the cortical bone but also of spongy bone. It is extremely efficient.
- A cone pin is inserted to determine the right axis.
- IM2: cutting insert with internal irrigation. This insert determines the 2-mm-diameter pilot osteotomy.
- Parallel pin.
- OT4: diamond-coated cone insert for differential preparation of the alveolar space inside the pilot osteotomy, i.e., to correct the axis and move the preparation before the final insert.

- IM3: 3-mm-diameter sharp insert with dual irrigation.
- Tapper: any cortical bone over 1 mm is tapped with a bur of the same system of the implant that is to be placed.

10.2 Surgical Technique

Correct execution of the surgical technique entails preoperative anaylsis of each implant site. Their measurements are recorded in a clinical file describing the quantity and quality of bone necessary for decision making using a new bone classification developed by the author.

Correct execution of implant site preparation with Mectron-Piezosurgery® requires adequate skill in performing basic techniques with ultrasonic instruments and specific training in bone perforation techniques.

Surgical skills are indispensable to apply the right amount of pressure on the handle, which leads to major intra-operatory benefits, such as increased control and sensitivity compared to micromotors.

Table 10.1 Clinical advantages of using Mectron-Piezosurgery® in Ultrasonic Implant Site Preparation

SURGICAL TECHNIQUE	LIMITS OF TRADITIONAL INSTRUMENTS	ADVANTAGES USING PIEZOSURGERY
1. Thin crest	Mandible implant site preparation using twist drills often results in buccal dehiscence.	Preparation of the implant site using Mectron-Piezosurgery® does not cause any dehiscence even when the crest is thin. Preparation of the pilot osteotomy can be optimized by using the diamond-coated insert (OT4) making it possible to reduce the thickness of the lingual cortical bone from the inside. The author named this technique "differential preparation of the implant site".
2. Soft bone	When the spongy bone is not very dense, the vibrations generated by a twist drill fracture osseous trabeculae around the site.	The microvibrations generated when using Mectron-Piezosurgery® conserves the integrity of the trabeculae in and around the implant site.
3. Proximity of alveolar nerve	Preparation of the site with the twist drill, where there is mineralized bone, requires strong pressure on the handle (about 2 kg). This reduces surgical control and increases the risk of neural damage.	When there is mineralized bone, preparation of the implant site using Mectron-Piezosurgery® requires light pressure on the handle (about 500 g). Surgical control is excellent, especially when the perforation of the last 2 mm in the proximity of the alveolar nerve is performed with a diamond-coated insert. The risk of neural damage is reduced considerably and only happens when the technique or instruments are not used correctly.

SURGICAL TECHNIQUE	LIMITS OF TRADITIONAL INSTRUMENTS	ADVANTAGES USING PIEZOSURGERY
4. Sinus Lift	The sinus lift technique for implant purposes can be performed in one or two operations. This depends on the ability to obtain enough primary stability of the implants. The crest height is generally a minimum of 4 mm when using burs.	Preparation of the implant site using Mectron-Piezosurgery® makes it possible to ensure sufficient primary stability for the implant even when the crest thickness is 2-3 mm. Placing the implants in the same surgical procedure as the sinus lift is a great advantage for both the patient and the surgeon performing the operation.
5. Intra-alveolar preparation	Preparation of the implant site does not always follow natural inclination of the alveolus. The result is that it is necessary to create a surgical alveolus inside the natural alveolus. This change in direction is difficult to obtain with a 2 mm twist drill since it mainly cuts on the tip.	Mectron-Piezosurgery's IM1 insert makes it very easy to change direction of the surgical alveolus with respect to the natural one. Subsequent use of the IM2 and OT4 makes it possible to optimize implant placement according to prosthesis priorities.
6. Osseous integration process	The process of osseous integration requires about two months to obtain secondary stability when ridged surface implants are used.	Initial bio-molecular and histomorphometric studies comparing Mectron-Piezosurgery and the twist drill on the same type of implant surface have demonstrated much faster bone healing in sites prepared with ultrasound.[77]
7. Immediate loading	Immediate loading depends on the resistance of primary stability prior to secondary stability. The favorable results depend on: bone characteristics, implant characteristics, implant site preparation.	The immediate loading technique using ultrasonic surgery makes the procedure more predictable. The anatomical characteristics can be exploited to achieve primary stability. In addition, bone healing is faster, especially in post-extraction.

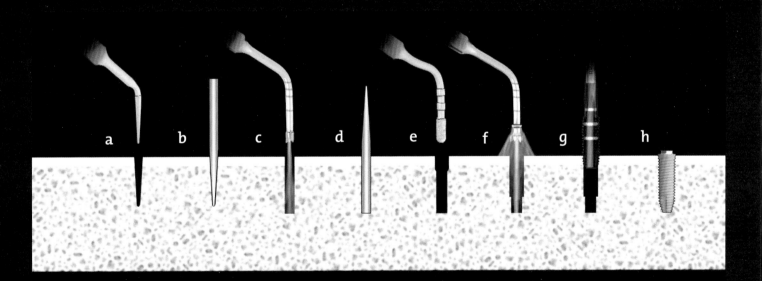

a) IM1 begins bone perforation. The maximum diame-
    ter of the cone-shaped insert is 2 mm.
b) First parallel pin.
c) IM2 produces the pilot osteotomy. The difference in
    mineralization between the cortical and spongy
    bone can be seen during the bone cutting action.
    The cylinder-shaped insert of the sharp tip and

the author enables specific work on several walls in
the pilot osteotomy to correct the implant axis. This
2.4-mm-diameter cylindrical diamond-coated insert
requires little pressure on the handle and it has
abundant irrigation.

f) IM3: for final preparation of the implant site for 4-
    mm-diameter implants. This insert has a sharp crown

CASE I

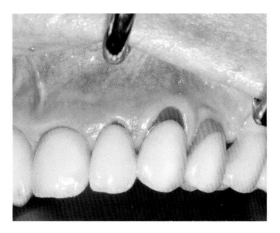

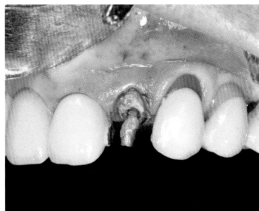

FIG 10-01 Initial photo of the lateral incisor that needs extracting.

FIG 10-02 Tooth lost due to root decay.

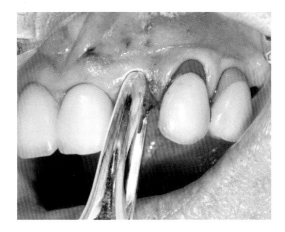

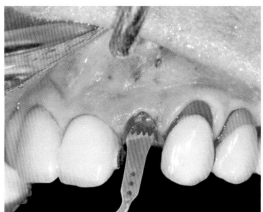

FIG 10-03 The mobility required for extraction cannot be obtained with manual instruments.

FIG 10-04 OT7 is used to perform a mesiodistal root fraction.

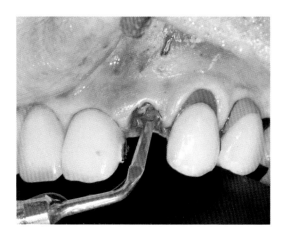

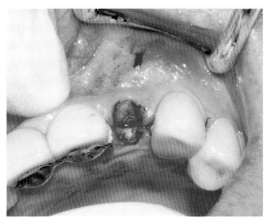

FIG 10-05 The root resection is performed until reaching the apex.

FIG 10-06 Occlusal view.

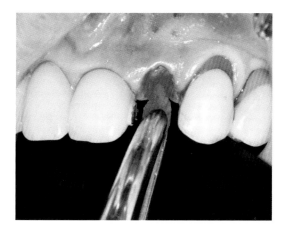

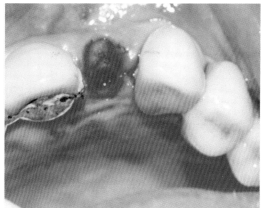

FIG 10-07 Removal of the apical fragment.

FIG 10-08 The buccal fragment is extracted in the palatinal direction without touching the buccal alveolar bone.

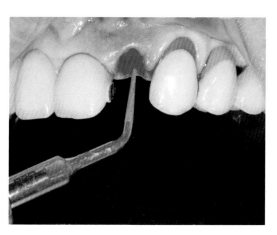

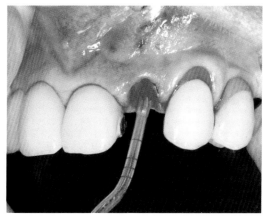

FIG 10-09 Insert IM1 is used to perform the initial pilot osteotomy.

FIG 10-10 Insert IM2 is used to perform the pilot osteotomy in a slightly palatinal direction with respect to the natural alveolus.

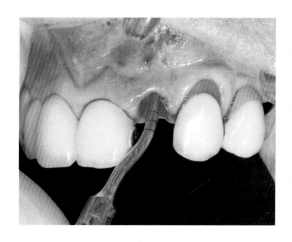

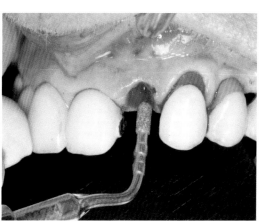

FIG 10-11 The pilot osteotomy is deepened using the depth indicators.

FIG 10-12 Insert OT4 is used to finalize the implant site.

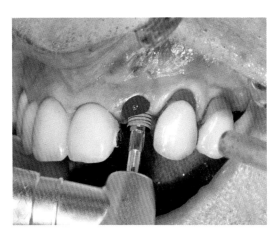

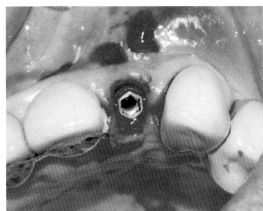

FIG 10-13 The cone implant is inserted.

FIG 10-14 Occlusal view of implant preparation in the correct position.

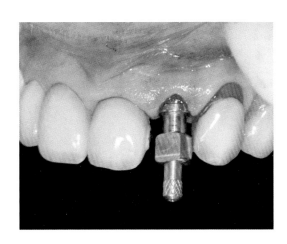

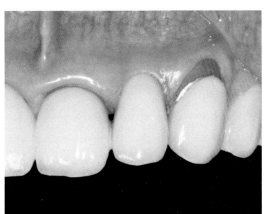

FIG 10-15 The transfer for impression.

FIG 10-16 Prosthesis crown performed by Dr. Cesare Robello and the dental technician Alberto Rovegno.

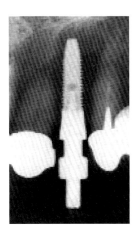

FIG 10-17 Radiographic control of correct implant position.

CASE II

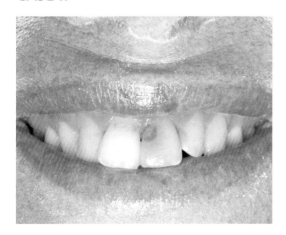

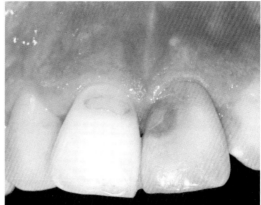

FIG 10-18 Destructive decay in central upper-left incisor: notice the high smile line with the upper lip near the gingival edge.

FIG 10-19 The extensive decay does not enable conservative recovery.

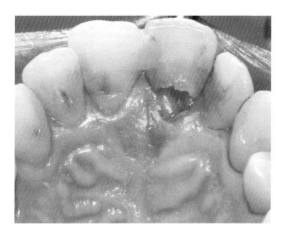

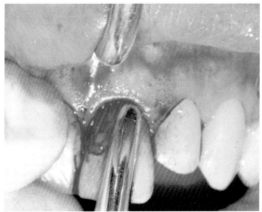

FIG 10-20 The cavity hits the root underneath the periodontal tissue: the tooth is lost.

FIG 10-21 The tooth crown is extracted with a traditional technique.

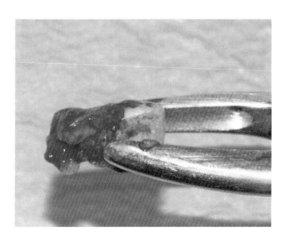

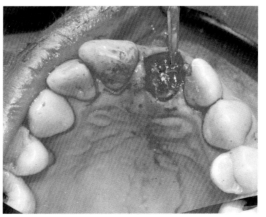

FIG 10-22 Notice the inflamed tissue on the decayed tooth base.

FIG 10-23 Insert EX1 is used for mesial-distal root fractioning.

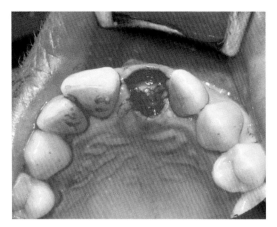

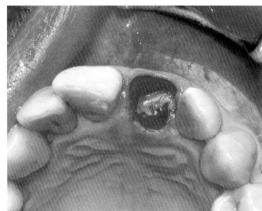

FIG 10-24 The palatinal fragment of the root is removed.

FIG 10-25 The root is pushed in a palatinal direction without touching the buccal wall of the alveolus.

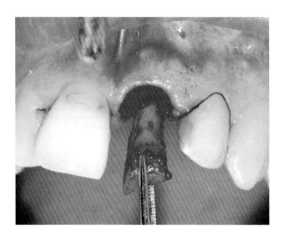

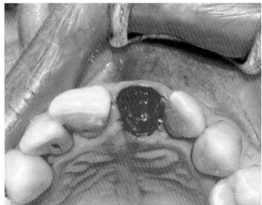

FIG 10-26 The root is extracted while keeping all the alveolar walls intact.

FIG 10-27 Insert PS2 is used to remove the inflamed tissue and the gutta-percha from the apical region.

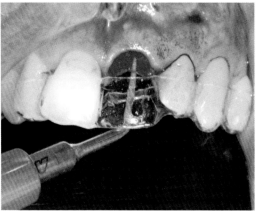

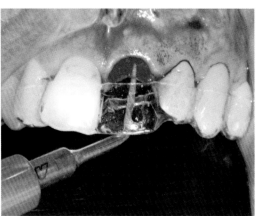

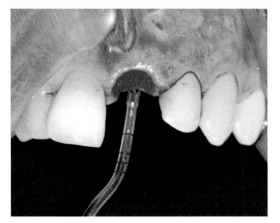

FIG 10-28 Insert IM1 is used to start differential preparation of the implant site in the alveolus. A surgical template is used for three-dimensional control.

FIG 10-29 Insert IM2 is used to perform the pilot osteotomy in a slightly palatinal direction with respect to the natural alveolus.

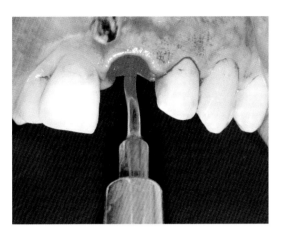

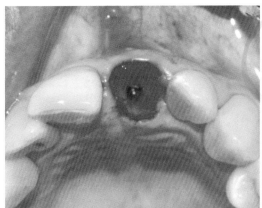

FIG 10-30 Insert IM2 is implemented until reaching the cortical of the nasal floor. Intraoperatory sensitivity is high thanks to the microvibration characteristics of Mectron-Piezosurgery®.

FIG 10-31 At first the pilot osteotomy appears correct in the buccal-palatinal dimension but in a position that is slightly mesial with respect to the alveolar apex.

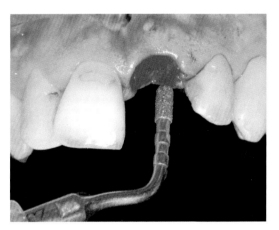

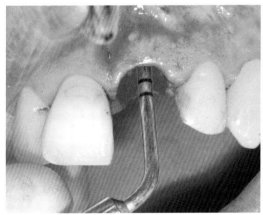

FIG 10-32 The diamond-coated insert OT4 is used for differential preparation inside the pilot osteotomy to finalize the implant site.

FIG 10-33 It is now possible to notice the optimal position of the hole after assessing the axis of the preparation with a parallel pin.

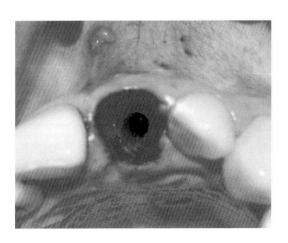

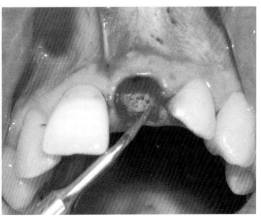

FIG 10-34 Final view of the endo-alveolar preparation of the implant site with IM3.

FIG 10-35 The bone stimulation technique, developed by the author, is implemented using insert OP5. By perforating the width of the hard plate, bleeding is stimulated in the spongy bone area in order to increase peri-implant vascular contribution.

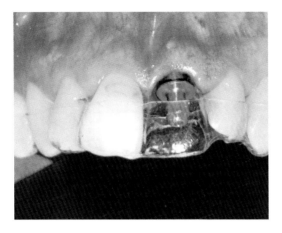
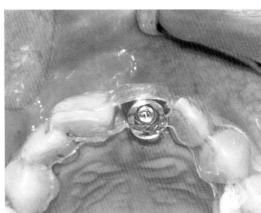

FIG 10-36 and FIG 10-37 Three dimensional check to ensure the position of the implant is correct.

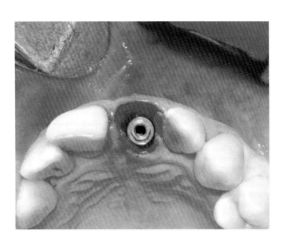
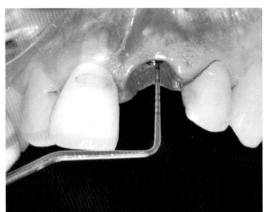

FIG 10-38 The correct position of the implant with respect to the bone walls and soft tissue.

FIG 10-39 Measuring the depth of the implant placed with respect to the height of the bone crest and gingival margin.

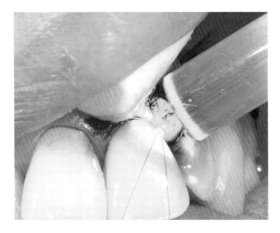
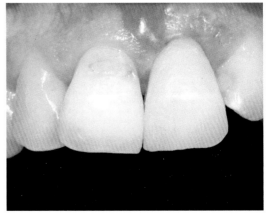

FIG 10-40 Positioning of the provisional crown and suture stitches stabilized with composite according to the Homa Zadeh technique.

FIG 10-41 Temporary crown after a year in operation.

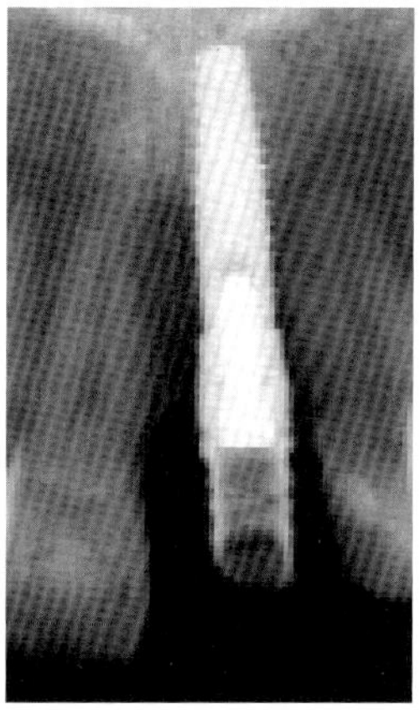

FIG 10-42 Notice the presence of newly formed bone around the implant head.

Orthodontic Microsurgery: New Corticotomy Technique

11

In adult patients, characterized by higher crest bone mineralization, traditional orthodontal movement also happens by activating a sort of periodontal tissue stress followed by the bone reabsorption necessary for tooth movement. Unfortunately, from a clinical standpoint, it is not always possible to apply to each tooth the right force required for movement.

A common consequence is that tissue resistance results in excessive compression of periodontal ligament fibers. In this way, the situation inadvertently passes from physiology to pathology. Lesions found in the inner periodontium are difficult to diagnose. A radiographic test shows only root apical resorption. This is the case in 90% of adult patients undergoing orthodontic treatment.[26,29,32,33,36,40,54,63,76]

In order to reduce osseous resistance in the direction of tooth movement and to reduce the length of treatment, some authors have proposed using surgery to facilitate tooth movement.[28] With these surgical techniques, traditional tooth movement is faster and has a lower risk of root resorption, which can be diagnosed with a radiograph.

11.1 New Surgically Guided Dental Movement

Drawing from these techniques, the author, in collaboration with the orthodontist Dr. Andrea Podestà, developed a new method for tooth movement which further decreases the risk of periodontal lesions. This new method, called "The Monocortical Tooth Dislocation (MTD) and Ligament Distraction (LD) Technique", is characterized by dislocation of the tooth and cortical bone in the direction of movement and a rapid distraction of the ligament on the opposite root surface.[76] This new technique, called Orthodontic Microsurgery, has the advantage that it is minimally invasive but very effective when performed with precision from a surgical and bio-mechanical standpoint.

11.2 Surgical Technique

The Corticotomy

The surgical technique used for MTD and LD consists of performing a perioradicular corticotomy of the bone surface in the direction of movement. For dental expansion, a corticotomy is performed to break the integrity of the buccal cortical bone.

Choosing the right surgical technique for each patient requires preoperative analysis carried out with periapical radiographs, which makes it possible to accurately establish osteotomy shape, according to the tooth movement required. In particular, it is important to assess the mesio-distal thickness of the adjacent tooth and the position of the radicular apex.[76]

This technique is based on the precision of bone cutting with respect to the root surfaces.

Surgical Instruments

Knowledge of the features of the Mectron-Piezosurgery® microsaw, developed to perform this technique, is extremely important in order to prevent root lesions and to obtain quicker dental movement. OT7S inserts, which belong to a special series for surgeons with experience in piezoelectric surgery, are characterized by their width of 0.35 mm and small size, with enabling them to meet anatomical needs. The main terminal is OT7S with four teeth, which can be accompanied by the smaller one with three teeth.

The bone is cut by using the vertical surface of the insert. This general rule becomes absolute when near or in contact with the root surace. In the crown portion, the corticomy is terminated with a joint cut needed to preserve the top of the interproximal bone.

11.3 Clinical Advantages using Piezosurgery in Orthodontic Microsurgery

The Monocortical Tooth Dislocation (MTD) and Ligament Distraction Technique (LDT) is a new method of tooth movement in adult patients that prevents lesions in periodontal tissues and reduces average treatment time by two-thirds. This movement, like others that belong to orthodontic microsurgery, conceived by the author, is only possible thanks to the Mectron-Piezosurgery® cutting characteristics using dedicated inserts. An outline comparing Mectron-Piezosurgery® to traditional instruments is not possible, because traditional instruments do not enable obtaining results that are at the base of dental dislocation movement.

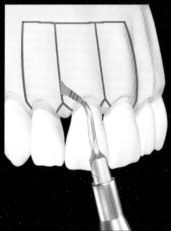

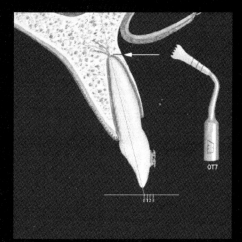

Orthodontic microsurgery: a periradicular corticotomy is performed on the bone surface found
in the direction of planned dental movement.
The vertical incisions are made at the center of
the interproximal bone while the horizontal
incision is made 4-5 mm higher than the root
apex. The discharge incisions make it possible to
preserve the interproximal bone.

Using insert OT7 it is possible to perform a horizontal bone cut also in the vicinity of the root
apex. In these cases, it is important to limit the
depth of the cut to only the width of the cortical
bone.

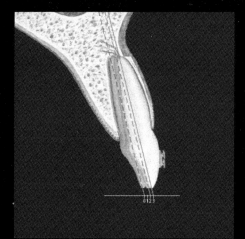

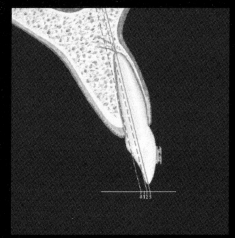

The biomechanical force applied to each tooth
produces new tooth movement:
• Monocortical tooth dislocation in the direction
  of movement.
• Rapid ligament distraction in the opposite
  direction of movement.

After completing movement, bone healing does
not change the width of the buccal cortical
bone. Bone healing also stabilizes the tooth
movement obtained, thereby simplifying the
containment period after treatment.

CASE I

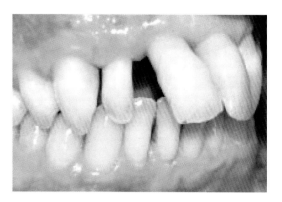
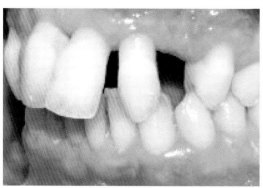

FIG 11-01 Class I relationship with anterior pathologic diastema in the right maxilla.

FIG 11-02 Class I molar and Class II canine relationship with absence of lateral incisors and diastema in the left maxilla.

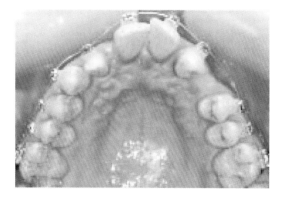
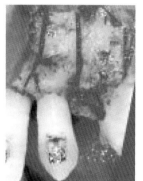

FIG 11-03 Day 0: after indirect bonding.

FIG 11-04 A vertical "Y" corticotomy is performed to preserve interproximal bone.

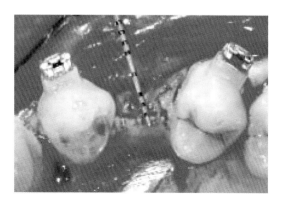
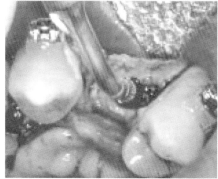

FIG 11-05 Edentulous ridge with insufficient width for implant positioning. A horizontal osteotomy for the ridge expansion technique is performed.

FIG 11-06 The piezosurgery OT4 insert is used to perform the differential implant site preparation technique.

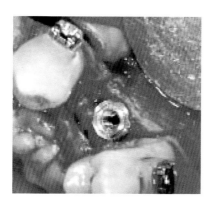 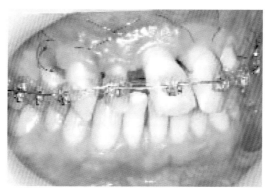

FIG 11-07 A 4-mm-diameter implant is placed in the expanded ridge.

FIG 11-08 The postoperative period was characterized by low morbidity; soft tissue quality was good at the time of suture removal.

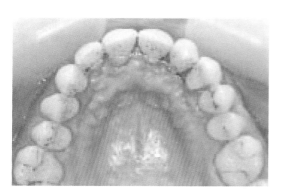 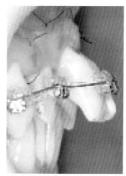 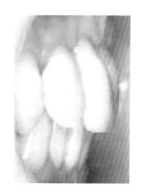

FIG 11-09 Day 63: Completion of therapy. A provisional crown has been placed on the maxillary left canine implant.

FIG 11-10 Initial overjet.

FIG 11-11 Final overjet.

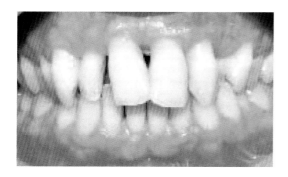 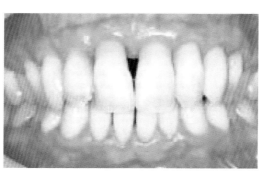

FIG 11-12 Malocclusion prior to treatment.

FIG 11-13 The final result 63 days later.

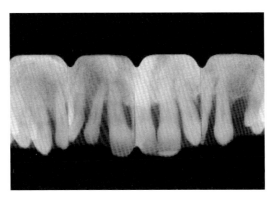
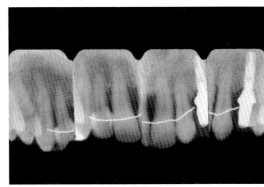

FIG 11-14 Radiograph at 3 months after MTDLD treatment.

FIG 11-15 Radiograph at 3 months after MTDLD treatment.

CASE II

FIG 11-16 Pre-surgery examination: lower-incisor crowding. Soft tissue assessment: to perform orthodontic microsurgery techniques the periodontal tissues must be healthy or treated.

FIG 11-17 After lifting the flap completely the root surface is cleansed using the diamond-coated OP5 insert and setting the device to „Root" mode.

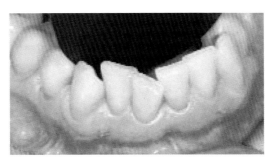
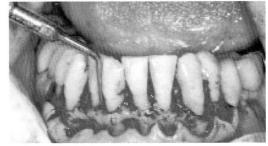

FIG 11-18 The root is smoothened using the smooth surface PP1 insert.

FIG 11-19 Notice the glossiness of the smoothened root surfaces.

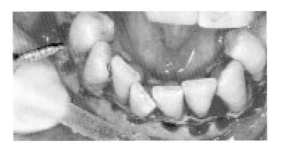
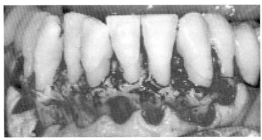

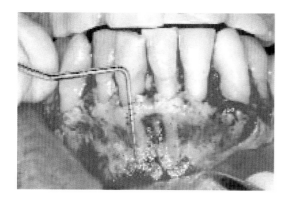

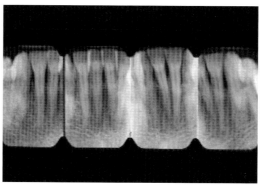

FIG 11-20 The periodontal probe is used to relate the radiographic length of the roots to the topographic anatomy .

FIG 11-21 Periapical XR for presurgical study.

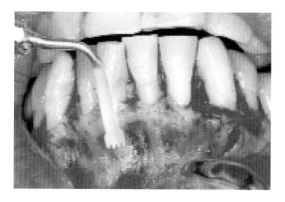

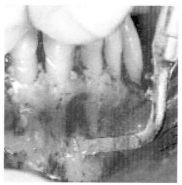

FIG 11-22 Insert OT7S is characterized by its small size: the blade has only 4 teeth and it is only 0.35 mm thick. The device should be set on "Special" mode when using this insert.

FIG 11-23 The corticotomy is begun by making vertical incisions in an apex-coronal direction.

FIG 11-24 The vertical incision near the interproximal bone crest should be in the shape of a "Y" in order to perform 2 discharge incisions which preserve the tip of the interproximal bone. Notice the correct position of the insert, which is able to touch the root surface with the vertical part and never with the sharp part of the saw.

FIG 11-25 The horizontal corticotomy is performed about 4-6 mm from the tooth apex. The depth of the cut must just slightly pass the cortical width.

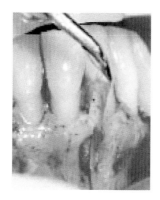

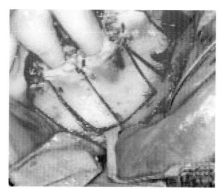

FIG 11-26 Corticotomies after the operation: notice the total preservation of cortical mineralization of each root.

FIG 11-27 5-0 suture with interrupted stitches.

FIG 11-28, 11-29, 11-30 After surgery is terminated indirect bandaging is applied immediately: notice enamel preparation with phosphoric acid (courtesy of Dr. A. Podestà).

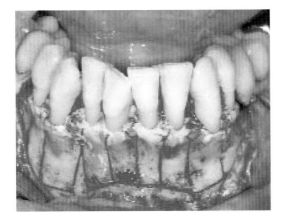
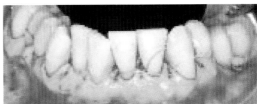
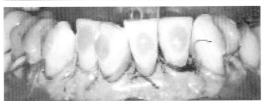

FIG 11-31 Indirect bandaging technique (courtesy of Dr. A. Podestà).

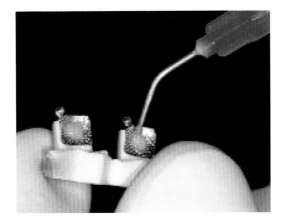
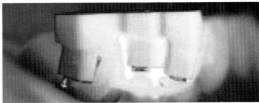
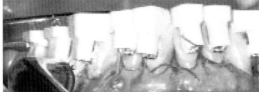

FIG 11-32 Bio-mechanic force is applied immediately after surgery (courtesy of Dr. A. Podestà).

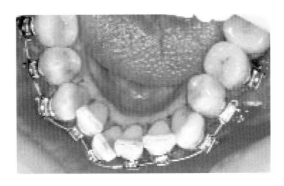

References

1. American Academy of Periodontology. Glossary of periodontal terms. 4th ed. Chicago, 2001.

2. Aro, Aho K, Kellokumpu-Lehtinen. Ultrasonic device in Bone Cutting. A Histological and Scanning Electron Microscopical Study. Acta Orthop Scand 1981; 52: 5–10.

3. Barone A, Santini S, Marconcini S, Giacomelli L, Gherlone E, Covani U. Osteotomy and membrane elevation during the maxillary sinus augmentation procedure. A comparative study: piezoelectric device vs. conventional rotative instruments. Clin Oral Implants Res. 2008 May;19(5):511–5.

4. Beziat JL, Vercellotti T, Gleizal A. Qu'est-ce que la Piezosurgery? Intérêt en Chirurgie cranio-maxillofaciale. A propos de deux ans d'expérience. (What is Piezosurgery?, Two-years experience in craniomaxillofacial surgery). Revue de Stomatologie et Chir Maxillofaciale, 2007; 108(2): 101–107.

5. Beziat JL, Béra,JC, Lavandier B, Gleizal A. Ultrasonic osteotomy as a new technique in craniomaxillofacial surgery. International Journal of Maxillo-facial Surgery, 2007; 36(6): 493–500.

6. Boioli LT, Vercellotti T, Tecucianu JF. La chirurgie piézoélectrique: Une alternative aux techniques classiques de chirurgie osseuse. Inf Dent 2004; 86 (41): 2887–2893.

7. Boioli LT, Etrillard P, Vercellotti T, Tecucianu JF. Piézochirurgie et aménagement osseux préimplantaire. Greffes par apposition de blocs d'os autogène avec prélèvement ramique. Implant 2005; 11(4): 261–274.

8. Boyne PJ, James RA. Grafting of the maxillary sinus floor with autogenous marroe and bone. J. Oral Surg 1980;38:613–616.

9. Cipriano L, Cimmino R, De Paolis G, Guerra F, Pillon A, Caputo M, et al. Piezosurgery mandibular enostosis: case report. G Chir 2007 May; 28(5):222–6.

10. Eggers G, Klein J, Blank J, Hassfeld S. Piezosurgery: an ultrasound device for cutting bone and its use and limitations in maxillofacial surgery. British Journal of Oral Maxillofacial Surgery. 2004; 42(5):451–3.

11. Friedman N. Periodontal Osseous surgery: Osteoplasty and Ostectomy. J Periodontol. 1995; 26:257–63.

12. Gargiulo AW, Wentz FM, Orban B, Dimensions and relations of the dentogingival junction in humans. J Periodontol 1961; 32: 261–7.

13. Geha H, Gleizal A, Nimeskern N, Beziat JL. Sensitivity of the Inferior Lip and Chin following Mandibular Bilateral Sagittal Split Osteotomy Using Piezosurgery. Plast. Reconstr. Surg. 2006; 118(7): 1598–1607.

14. Gleizal A, Béra JC, Lavandier B., Béziat JL. Piezoelectric osteotomy: a new technique for bone surgery - advantages in craniofacial surgery. Childs Nerv Syst. 2007; 23(5): 509–513.

15. Gleizal A, Béra JC, Lavandier B., Béziat JL. Craniofacial approach for orbital tumors and ultrasonic bone cutting. J Fr Ophtalmol. 2007 Nov;30(9):882–91.

16. González-García A, Diniz-Freitas M, Somoza-Martín M, García-García A. Piezoelectric Bone Surgery Applied in Alveolar Distraction Osteogenesis: A Technical Note. Int J Oral Maxillofac Implants 2007;22:1012–1016.

17. Grenga V, M. Bovi. Piezoelectric Surgery for Exposure of Palatally Impacted Canines. Journal of Clinical Orthodontics. 2004; Volume 38(8): 446–448.

18. Gruber RM, Kramer FJ, Merten HA, Schliephake H. Ultrasonic surgery – an alternative way in orthognathic surgery of the mandible. A pilot study. Int. J. of Oral Maxillofacial Surg. 2005; 34: 590–593.

19. Guo ZZ, Liu X, Li Y, Deng YF, Wang Y. The use of Piezosurgery osteotomy in treatment of longstanding maxillary fractures: report of 12 consecutive patients. Shangai Kou Qiang Yi Xue. 2007 Feb;16(1):97–9.

20. Happe A. Use of Piezoelectric Surgical Device to Harvest Bone Grafts from the Mandibular Ramus: Report of 40 cases. Int J Periodontics Restorative Dent. 2007; 27(3): 240–249.

21. Horton JE, Tarpley TM Jr, Wood LD. The healing of surgical defects in alveolar bone produced with ultrasonic instrumentation, chisel, and rotary bur. Oral Surg Oral Med Oral Phat-1975; 39(4):536–546.

22. Horton JE, Tarpley TM Jr, Jacoway JR. Clinical Applications of Ultrasonic Instrumentation in the Surgical Removal Bone. Oral Surg Oral Med Oral Pathol 1981; 51: 236–242.

23. Kois J. The restorative-periodontal interface: biological parameters. Periodontology 2000. 1996; 11: 29–38.

24. Kotrikova B, Wirtz R, Krempien R, Blank J, Eggers G, Samiotis A, et al. Piezosurgery –a new safe technique in cranial osteplasty, Int J Oral Maxillofacial Surgery. 2006 May; 35(5):461–5.

25. Kramer FJ, Ludwig HC, Materna T, Gruber R, Marten HA, Shliephake H. Piezoelectric osteotomies in craniofacial procedures: a series of 15 pediatric patients. J Neurosurg (1 Suppl Pediatrics) 2006, 104: 68–71.

26. Kuijpers - Jagtman AM. Treatment - related factors for external root resorption during orthodontic treatment. 10. American Association of Orthodontists – Annual Session, Seattle, 2007.

27. Lambrecht JT. Intraorale Piezo-Chirurgie. Schweiz Monatsschr Zahnmed. 1/2004; 114: 29–36.

28. Norton LA, Burstone CJ. The biophysics of bone remodeling during orthodontics-optimal force considerations. In Raton B. The Biology of Tooth Movement. Fla:CRC Press; 1989:321–334.

29. Mazorow HB. Bone repair after experimental produced defects. J Oral Surg 1960; 18: 107–115.

30. McFall TA, Yamane GM, Burnett GW. Comparison of the cutting effect on bone of an ultrasonic cutting device and rotary burs. J Oral Surg, Anesth & Hosp D Serv 1961; 19: 200–209.

31. McLaughlin RP, Bennett JC, Trevisi H. Meccaniche Ortodontiche: Un Approccio Sistematico (Systemized Orthodontic Treatment Mechanics). Mosby International Ltd., 2001 336.

32. Oppenheim A. Human tissue response to orthodontic intervention of short and long duration. Am J Orthod Oral Surg. 1942;28:263–301.

33. Peivandi A, Bugnet R, Debize E, Gleizal A, Dohan DM. Piezoelectric osteotomy: applications in periodontal and implant surgery. Rev Stomatol Chir Maxillofac. 2007 Nov;108(5):431–440.

34. Pontoriero R, Carnevale G. Surgical Crown Lengthening: A 12- month clinical wound healing study. J Periodontol. 2001; 72:841–8.

35. Proffit WR, Fields HW Jr, Moray LJ. Malocclusion prevalence and orthodontic treatment need in the U.S.A. estimates from NHANES III survej. Int J Orthodon Orthognat Surgery 1998;13(2):97–106.

36. Proffit WR. Contemporary Orthodontics. St Louis, Calif: Mosby-Year Book Inc, 1999; 296–325.

37. Quinn RS, Yoshikawa K. A reassessment of force magnitude in orthodontics. Am J Orthod. 1985;88:252–260.

38. Reitan K. Clinical and histologic observations on tooth movement during and after orthodontic treatment. Am J Orthod. 1967;53:721–745.

39. Ren Y, Maltha JC, Kuijpers - Jagtman AM. Optimum Force Magnitude for Orthodontic Tooth Movement: A Systematic Literature Review. The Angle Orthodontist. Feb. 2002;73(1):86–92.

40. Robiony M, Polini F, Costa F, Vercellotti T, Politi M. Piezoelectric Bone Cutting in multipiece maxillary osteotomies. Technical Note. J Oral Maxillofac Surg. 2004;62:759–761.

41. Robiony M, Polini F, Costa F, Toro C, Politi M. Ultrasound Piezoelectric Vibrations to Perform Osteotomies in Rhinoplasty. Elsevier Ltd in Journal of Oral and Maxillofacial Surgery. 2007; 65(5): 1035–1038.

42. Robiony M, Polini F, Costa F, Zerman N, Politi M. Ultrasonic bone cutting for surgically assisted rapid maxillary expansion (SARME) under local anaesthesia. Int J Oral Maxillofac Surg. 2007; 36(3): 267–9.

43. Rosenberg ES, Cho SC, Garber DA. Crown lengthening revisited. Compend Contin Educ Dent. 1999; 20:527–32.

44. Sakkas N, Otten JE, Gutwald R, Schmelzeisen R. Transposition of the mental nerve by Piezosurgery followed by postoperative neurosensory control: A case report. Br J Oral Maxillofac Surg. 2007 Aug 9; [Epub ahead of print].

45. Schaeren S, Jaquiéry C, Heberer M, Tolnay M, Vercellotti T, Martin I. Assessment of Nerve Damage using a novel ultrasonic device for bone cutting. Journal of Oral and Maxillofacial Surgery 66: 593–596, 2008.

46. Schaller BJ, Gruber R, Merten HA, Kruschat T, Schliephake H, Buchfelder M, et al. Piezoelectric bone surgery: a revolutionary technique for minimally invasive surgery in cranial base and spinal surgery? Neurosurgery. Technical notes. 2005; Operative Neurosurgery 57: suppl. 4.

47. Schlee M. Ultraschallgestutzte Chirurgie – Grundlagen und Moglichkeiten. Zeitschrift fur Zahnärztliche Implantologie (JDI) 2005; 21. Jahrgang, Heft 1 (2005) Seite 48–59.

48. Sembronio S, Albiero AM, Polini F, Robiony M, Politi M. Intraoral endoscopically assisted treatment of temporomandibular joint ankylosis: Preliminary report. Oral Surg Oral Med Oral Pathol Oral Radiol Endod. 2007 May 10.

49. Siervo S, Ruggli-Milic S, Radici M, Siervo P, Jäger K. Piezoelectric surgery. An alternative method of minimally invasive surgery. Schweiz Monatsschr Zahnmed. 2004; 114(4): 365–377.

50. Sivolella S, Berengo M, Scarin M, Mella F, Martinelli F. Autogenous particulate bone collected with a piezo-electric surgical device and bone trap: a microbiological and histomorphometric study. Archives of Oral Biology. 2006; 51(10): 883–891.

51. Sivolella S, Berengo M, Fiorot M, Mazzuchin M. Retrieval of blade implants with Piezosurgery: two clinical cases. Minerva Stomatol. 2007 Jan-Feb;56(1-2):53–61.

52. Smukler H, Chaibi M, Periodontal and dental considerations in clinical crown extension: A rational basis for treatment. Int J Periodontics Rest Dent. 1997; 17:465–77.

53. Storey E, Smith R. Force in orthodontics and its relation to tooth movement. Aust Dent J. 1952;56:11–18.

54. Stubinger S, Robertson A, Zimmerer SK, Leiggener C, Sader R, Kunz C. Piezoelectric Harvesting of an Autogenous Bone Graft from the Zygomaticomaxillary Region: Case Report. Int J Periodontics Restorative Dent. 2006; 26(5): 453–457.

55. Stubinger S., Goethe J.W. Bone Healing After Piezosurgery and its Influence on Clinical Applications. Journal of Oral and Maxillofacial Surgery, Volume 65, Issue 9, Pages 39.e7–39.e8.

56. Stübinger S, Landes C, Seitz O, Zeilhofer HF, Sader R. Ultrasonic Bone Cutting in oral Surgery: a Review of 60 cases [Article in German]. Ultraschall Med. 2008 Feb;29(1): 66–71.

57. Tatum OH. Maxillary sinus grafting for endosseous implants. Lectur, Alabama Implant Study Group, Annual Meeting. Birmingham AL, 1997.

58. Tordjman S, Boioli LT, Fayd N. Apport de la Piézochirurgie dans la surélévation du plancher sinusien. Dèpartement de Parodontologie de l'UFR de Stomatologie et Chirurgie Maxillo-Faciale. Universitè de Paris VI – Paris. Revue Implantologie – novembre 2006: 17–25.

59. Torella F, Pitarch J, Cabanes G, Anitua E. Ultrasonic Osteotomy for the Surgical Approach of the Maxillary Sinus: A technical note. Int J Oral Maxillofac Implants 1998; 13:697–700.

60. Troiani C, Russo C, Ballarani G, Vercellotti T. Piezoelectric Surgery: A new reality to cut and manage bone. Maxillo Odontostomatologia – International Journal of Maxillo Odontostomatology – S.I.M.O. 2005; 4(1): 23–28.

61. Valencia ME, Hernandez RM, Solange BV, Jaramillo KJ. Osteotomìas Piezoelèctricas en Cirugìa Ortognatica. Revista de la Facultad de Odontologia. Universidad de Valparaiso. 2004; 3: 693–695.

62. Verna CA, in Biomechanics in Orthodontics B.Melsen, G. Fiorelli software. See on www.libra-ortho.it.

63. Vercellotti T. Piezoelectric Surgery in Implantology: A Case Report – A New Piezoelectric Ridge Expansion Technique. Int J Periodontics Restorative Dent 2000; 20(4): 359–365.

64. Vercellotti T, Russo C, Gianotti S. A New Piezoelectric Ridge Expansion Technique in the Lower Arch – A Case Report (online article). World Dentistry 2000; http://www.worlddent.com/2001/05/articles/vercellotit.xml.

65. Vercellotti T, De Paoli S, Nevins M. The Piezoelectric Bony Window Osteotomy and Sinus Membrane Elevation: Introduction of a New Technique for Simplification of the Sinus Augmentation Procedure. Int J Periodontics Restorative Dent 2001; 21(6): 561–567.

66. Vercellotti T, Crovace A, Palermo A, Molfetta A. The Piezoelectric Osteotomy in Orthopedics: Clinical and Histological Evaluations (Pilot Study in Animals). Mediterranean Journal of Surg Med 2001; 9: 89–95.

67. Vercellotti T, Obermair G. Introduction to Piezosurgery®. Dentale Implantologie & Parodontologie. 2003; 7: 270–274.

68. Vercellotti T. La Chirurgia Ossea Piezoelettrica. Il Dentista Moderno. 2003; 5: 21–55.

69. Vercellotti T. Technological characteristics and clinical indications of piezoelectric bone surgery. Minerva Stomatol. 2004; 53(5): 207–14.

70. Vercellotti T. Caracterìsticas tecnològicas e indicaciones clìnicas de la cirugìa òsea piezoeléctrica. Revista Mundo Dental. 2005; 26–28.

71. Vercellotti T, Obermair G. Introduzione alla Chirurgia Piezoelettrica®. Implantologia Dentale. 2005; 2(2):78–82.

72. Vercellotti T. La Chirurgia piezoelettrica. Tecniche di rialzo del Seno Mascellare. In Testori T, Weinstein R, Wallace S. La Chirurgia del Seno Mascellare e le alternative terapeutiche. Gorizia: Edizioni Acme 2005; 14:245–255.

73. Vercellotti T, Nevins ML, Kim DM, Nevins M, Wada K, Schenk RK, et al. Osseous Response following Resective Therapy with a Piezosurgery®. Int J Periodontics Restorative Dent. 2005; 25(6): 543–549.

74. Vercellotti T, Pollack AS. The New Bone Surgery Device: Sinus Grafting and Periodontal Surgery. Compend Contin Educ Dent. 2006 May;27(5): 319–25.

75. Vercellotti T, Nevins M, Jensen Ole T. Piezoelectric Bone Surgery for Sinus Bone Grafting. In Jensen Ole T. The Sinus Bone Graft. Quintessence, 2006; 23: 273–279.

76. Vercellotti T, Podestà A. Orthodontic Microsurgery: A New Surgically Guided Technique for Dental Movement. Int J Periodontics Restorative Dent. 2007;27: 325–331.

77. Vercellotti T, Majzoub Z, Trisi P, Valente ML, Sabbini E, Cordioli G. Histologic Evaluation of Bone Response to Piezoelectric, Surgical Saw and Drill Osteotomies in the Rabbit Calvaria. The International Journal of Oral & Maxillofacial Implants (submitted).

78. Vercellotti T. The Piezoelectric Bone Surgery: New Paradigme. Quintessence Publisher.

79. Wallace SS, Froum SJ. Effect of maxillary sinus augmentation on the survival of endosseous dental implants. A systematic review. Ann Periodontol 2003;8:328–343.

80. Wallace SS, Mazor Z, Froum SJ, Sang-Choon Cho, Tarnow DP. Schneiderian Membrane Perforation Rate During Sinus Elevation Using Piezosurgery: Clinical Results of 100 Consecutive Cases. Int J Periodontics Restorative Dent. 2007 Sept/Oct;27(5).

81. Wilko WM, Wilko MT. Wilkodontics® Orthodontic System and the Accelerated Osteogenic Orthodontics™ Procedure Rapid Tooth Movement With Decortication and Alveolar Augmentation. J Period & Restorative Dentistry 2001;21:9–19.

Additional Literature

Bovi M. Mobilization of the Inferior Alveolar Nerve with simultaneous implant insertion: A New Technique. A Case Report. Int J Periodontics Restorative Dent 2005; 25(4): 375–383.

Blakenburg JJ, Both CJ, Borstlap WA, van Damme PA. Sound levels of the Piezosurgery. Risk of permanent damage to hearing. Ned Tijdschr Tandheelkd. 2007 Nov;114(11):451–4.

Bücking W. Empirisch in der Praxis bewahrt. Die schonende Explantation. Quintessenz. 2005; 56(4):335–341.

Chiriac G, Herten M, Schwarz F, Rothamel D, Becker J. Autogenous bone chips: influence of a new piezoelectric device (Piezosurgery®) on chips morphology, cell viability and differentiation. Journal of Clinical Periodontology 2005; 32:994–999.

Cortese G. Struttura implantare a nido d'ape per riabilitare selle atrofiche edentule posteriori. Un approccio chirurgico piezoelettrico. Teamwork. anno VI, 4/2004, 304–309.

D.J. Hoigne, S. Stübinger, O. Von Kaenel, S. Shamdasani, P. Hasenboehler. Piezoelectric osteotomy in hand surgery: first experiences with a new technique. BMC Musculoskeletal Disorders 2006; 7:36.

Enislidis G, Wittwer G, Ewers RDF. Preliminary Report on a Staged Ridge Slitting Technique for Implant Placement in the Mandible: A Technical note. Int J Oral Maxillofac Implants, 2006; 21: 445–449.

Gleizal A, Li Shuli, Pialat JB, Béziat JL. Transcriptional expression of calvarial bone after treatment with low - intensity ultrasound: An in vitro study. Ultrasound in Medicine & Biology 2006; 32(10): 1569–1574.

Maurer P, Kriwalsky MS, Block Veras R, Brandt J, Heiss C. Light microscopic examination of rabbit skulls following conventional and Piezosurgery osteotomy. Biomed Tech (Berl). 2007;52(5):351–5.

Preti G, Martinasso G, Peirone B, Navone R, Manzella C, Muzio G, et al. Cytokines and Growth Factors Involved in the Osseo-integration of Oral Titanium Implants Positioned using Piezoelectric Bone Surgery Versus a Drill Technique: A Pilot Study in Minipigs. Journal of Periodontology, 2007; 78(4): 716–722.

Robiony M, Toro C, Costa F, Sempronio S, Polini F, Politi T, Costa F. Piezosurgery: a new method for osteotomies in rhinoplasty. J Craniofacial Surgery. 2007 Sep; 18(5): 1098–100.

Robiony M, Polini F, Costa F, Sempronio S, Zerman N, Politi M. Endoscopically-Assisted Intraoral Vertical Ramus Osteotomy and Piezoelectric Surgery in Mandibular Prognathism. Int. J. Oral Maxillofac. Surg 2007 Oct ;65 (10):2119–24.

Salami A, Vercellotti T, Mora R, Dellepiane M. Piezoelectric Bone Surgery in otologic surgery. Otolaryngology – Head and Neck Surgery, 2007; 136: 484–485.

Salami A, Mora R, Dellepiane M Piezosurgery in the excision of middle-ear tumors: Effects on mineralized and non-mineralized tissues. Med Sci Monit. 2007 Dec; 13(12):PI25–29.

Salami A, Mora R, Dellepiane M. Piezosurgery in the exeresis of glomus tympanicum tumours. Eur Arch Othorinolaryngol. 2008 Jan 4 [Epub ahead of print].

Salami A, Dellepiane M, Mora F, Crippa B, Mora R. Piezosurgery® in the cochleostomy through multiple middle ear approaches. Int J Pediatr Otorhinolaryngol. 2008 May; 72(5):653–7.

Salami A, Dellepiane M, Mora R. A novel approach to facial nerve decompression: use of Piezosurgery(R). Acta Otolaryngol. 2008 May;128(5):530–3.

Tordjman S, Boioli LT, Fayd N. Apport de la Piézochirurgie dans la surélévation du plancher sinusien. Dèpartement de Parodontologie de l'UFR de Stomatologie et Chirurgie Maxillo-Faciale. Universitè de Paris VI. Paris. Revue Implantologie. novembre 2006: 17–25.

Vercellotti T, Dellepiane M, Mora R, Salami A. Piezoelectric Bone Surgery in otosclerosis. Acta Otolaryngol. 2007 Sep;127(9):932–7.

Accepted for publication

Robiony M, Polini F, Costa F, Sempronio S, Zerman N, Politi M. Endoscopically-Assisted Intraoral Vertical Ramus Osteotomy and Piezoelectric Surgery in Mandibular Prognathism. Elsevier Ltd in Int. J. Oral maxillofac. Surg.